编委会

主 编

邹云春　王　英　杨　必

副主编

范浩博　李柯然

编　委（以姓氏笔画为序）

王　英（川北医学院）　　　吕红彬（西南医科大学）
向倚弦（川北医学院）　　　邹云春（川北医学院）
李柯然（南京医科大学）　　张　磊（滨州医学院）
杨　必（四川大学）　　　　杨　桢（川北医学院）
宋雨桐（四川大学）　　　　范浩博（成都中医药大学）
罗　欧（川北医学院）　　　谭青青（川北医学院）

秘　书

向倚弦

Professional English for Optometry

眼视光学专业英语

主编

邹云春 王 英 杨 必

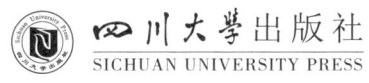

图书在版编目（CIP）数据

眼视光学专业英语 / 邹云春，王英，杨必主编. --成都：四川大学出版社，2025.1
ISBN 978-7-5690-6521-3

Ⅰ. ①眼… Ⅱ. ①邹… ②王… ③杨… Ⅲ. ①屈光学－英语－教材 Ⅳ. ①R778

中国国家版本馆CIP数据核字（2023）第254478号

书　　名：	眼视光学专业英语
	Yanshiguangxue Zhuanye Yingyu
主　　编：	邹云春　王　英　杨　必
选题策划：	许　奕
责任编辑：	余　芳
责任校对：	周　洁
装帧设计：	裴菊红
责任印制：	李金兰
出版发行：	四川大学出版社有限责任公司
地　　址：	成都市一环路南一段24号（610065）
电　　话：	（028）85408311（发行部）、85400276（总编室）
电子邮箱：	scupress@vip.163.com
网　　址：	https://press.scu.edu.cn
印前制作：	四川胜翔数码印务设计有限公司
印刷装订：	成都金阳印务有限责任公司
成品尺寸：	185 mm×260 mm
印　　张：	14.25
插　　页：	10
字　　数：	464千字
版　　次：	2025年1月 第1版
印　　次：	2025年1月 第1次印刷
定　　价：	79.00元

本社图书如有印装质量问题，请联系发行部调换

版权所有 ◆ 侵权必究

扫码获取数字资源

四川大学出版社
微信公众号

前　言

《眼视光学专业英语》是在我校视光学专业原自编英语教材《视光学概论》的基础上再次修订、更新而成。教材对版式进行了新的设计，提高了图片的清晰度，进一步提升了整体质量，增强了美感。

眼视光学专业的国际化发展趋势，要求未来的视光人才是具有国际视野和英语交流能力的全面发展的应用型专业技术人才。这要求眼视光学专业学子需具备自主学习、阅读英文医学文献资料，并与国际同行进行学术交流的能力。因此，专业英语教学已经成为眼视光教育的重要部分。目前，开设有眼视光学专业的全国各大医学院校基本都开设了专业英语课程，但缺乏符合我国视光教育实际情况的专门教材。

本书是学生学习《医学专业英语》之后，在眼视光学方向进行补充和提高的专业英语教材，着重从实用性角度出发，考虑到眼视光学专业学子未来岗位的实践性需求、学历提升以及科研发展需求，内容上侧重于眼视光学专业英语词汇、术语以及用法，同时融入了近年来眼视光学发展的新动态、新技术以及新方法，以帮助学生了解专业前沿，掌握专业发展动态，提高科研创新能力，增强自主学习、阅读和撰写英文文章的能力。

本书一共17章，第1章从验光的历史和范围出发，介绍了验光师和眼科医生的工作范畴，第2章介绍眼的解剖学、生理学特征，第3章至第8章介绍验光师工作的主要内容，即屈光不正及其常见临床检查、矫正方法，第9章至第16章介绍眼睛不同结构的疾病，第17章是情景教学资源和案例。

本书具有如下特点：

第一，每一章开始都有一个小节目录，展现了本章的组织架构，方便读者快速了解本章内容。各级标题和副标题、粗体字和斜体字有助于读者快速对主题进行定位。

第二，教材涵盖了眼视光学专业的基础内容，侧重专业英语词汇和用法表达，体现了眼视光学发展的新动态、新技术、新方法，可同时满足专业实践和科研需求，适合本科以及高职高专院校的视光学专业和眼视光医学专业使用。

第三，内容的选取考虑到职场环境下对英语的实际使用，是眼视光学专业学子在未来工作和学习中能真正派上用场的医学语料，以学以致用为目标，避免出现"学而不用"或"用而没学"的情况。

第四，新增较多临床案例图片和表格，生动、清晰地展示了相关知识，同时增强了可读性。

参与编写本教材的人员均为多年从事眼视光学和眼科学相关的教学或临床实践工作的专业技术人员，真诚地感谢团队的每一位成员在本书编撰成稿过程中付出的心血和努力。特别要真诚地感谢四川大学眼视光医学院的杨必教授、南京医科大学眼视光学系的李柯然教授、滨州医学院眼视光医学系的张磊教授、西南医科大学眼视光学系的吕红彬教授等人为本书相关章节的编写付出的辛勤劳动。

希望此书能够帮助广大眼视光学专业学子提高专业英语听、说、读、写的能力，推动眼视光学教育与国际接轨，提高眼视光人才培养的质量，培养出具有国际视野的、全面发展的应用型眼视光学人才。

尽管我们已经竭尽全力确保内容的准确性，但书中仍然有可能存在缺漏，因此，我们真诚希望读者能够对本书的内容积极探讨，指出不足之处，并给予我们反馈和建议。

邹云春

Contents

Chapter 1 Optometry 1

Chapter 2 Anatomy and Physiology of the Eye 4

Chapter 3 Clinic Methods in Optometry.. 21

Chapter 4 Refractive Error.. 34

Chapter 5 Optics & Refraction 50

Chapter 6 Accommodation and Vergence... 66

Chapter 7 Spectacles.. 79

Chapter 8 Contact Lenses 86

Chapter 9 Diseases of the Cornea 100

Chapter 10 Glaucoma 107

Chapter 11 Diseases of the Uveal Tract... 116

Chapter 12 Lens Diseases.. 130

Chapter 13 Retinal Diseases 150

Chapter 14 Strabismus and Nystagmus 168

Chapter 15 Low Vision and Vision Rehabilitation 181

Chapter 16 Binocular Vision... 197

Chapter 17 Common Clinical Conversations 204

Appendix... 221

Chapter 1
Optometry

INTRODUCTION
> ▶ Eye Problems
> ▶ Worldwide Careers

OPTOMETRIST AND OPHTHALMOLOGIST

1.1 INTRODUCTION

Optometry is a health care specialty, involving the eyes and their related structures, as well as human vision, visual system, and visual information processing.

Like most professions, optometry education, certification and practice are regulated in most countries. *Optometrists* and optometry related organizations interact with government agencies, other health care professionals and the community to provide eye and vision care. Optometry is one of the four major eye care specialties. Other specialties include *ophthalmology* (which is a branch of surgery), *opticians* and *orthopedics* (a subspecialty of ophthalmology mainly for the treatment of *strabismus*).

The word "optometry" comes from the Greek words *optos*, which means eye or vision, and *metria*, which means measurement.

The eye, including its structure and characteristics, has attracted scientists and the public since ancient times. Many expressions of understanding in English are equivalent visual terms. "I see" means "I understand".

1.1.1 Eye Problems

When told that they may have eye problems, many patients are more concerned about diseases affecting vision than other more fatal diseases. Blindness can have devastating psychological, economic and social effects, because many blind people need a lot of help in their daily activities of life and are often unable to continue the paid work they used to do.

Therefore, eye problems are often crucial.

The maintenance of eye health and the correction of eye problems with decreased vision greatly contribute to the understanding of the better life. In view of the importance of vision to the quality of life, many optometrists think their work is beneficial because they can often restore or improve the patient's vision.

Behavioural optometry is a related area of non-strabismus vision therapy that some optometrists practice. Generally, *ophthalmologists* do not practice this.

1.1.2 Worldwide Careers

In some countries such as the United States, optometrists have obtained from state legislatures the right to treat more eye conditions and to perform certain laser surgeries. Optometrists have been successful in getting the right to use some types of medication, depending on if the medication is given as pills, eye drops, or injections. In the United States, all states except for Oklahoma do not allow optometrists to perform any type of surgery. However, in Oklahoma, optometrists are allowed by the state legislature to perform *laser surgery*. While, In China, general optometrists have no prescription right. They usually do some *ophthalmic auxiliary examinations* in their daily work, or do sales, trainings, and management in companies. A few of them are teachers in some educational organizations. As the optometry developed, in 2012 the optometric medicine & ophthalmology was officially included in the undergraduate majors by the Ministry of Education. Qu Jia, who is the director of the national clinical research center for ocular diseases, is the first one that proposed the five-year optometry. After graduating from this major, students will have prescription rights with the title of optometric medicine doctor.

1.2 OPTOMETRIST AND OPHTHALMOLOGIST

Optometrists, also known as doctors of optometry, provide most primary vision care. They diagnose vision problems and eye diseases by examining people's eyes, and test patients' vision, depth, and color vision, as well as their ability to focus and coordinate their eyes. Optometrists can prescribe *eyeglasses* and *contact lenses* and provide *vision therapy* and *low-vision rehabilitation*. Optometrists analyze test results and develop a treatment plan. They give drugs to patients to help diagnose vision problems and prescribe drugs to treat some eye diseases. Optometrists usually provide preoperative and postoperative care for cataract patients and patients who have undergone laser vision correction or other ophthalmic surgery. They also diagnose conditions caused by systemic diseases such as diabetes and high blood pressure, referring patients to other health practitioners as needed.

Optometrists should not be confused with ophthalmologists or dispensing opticians. Ophthalmologists are physicians who perform eye surgery, as well as diagnose and treat eye diseases and injuries. Like optometrists, they also examine eyes and prescribe eyeglasses and contact lenses. Dispensing opticians fit and adjust eyeglasses and may also fit contact lenses according to prescriptions written by ophthalmologists or optometrists.

Most optometrists are in general practice. Some specialize in work with the elderly, children, or partially sighted persons who need specialized visual devices. Others develop and implement ways to protect workers' eyes from on-the-job strain or injury. Some specialize in contact lenses, sports vision, or vision therapy. A few teach optometry, perform research, or consult.

Most optometrists are private practitioners who handle the business aspects of running an office, such as developing a patient base, hiring employees, keeping paper and electronic records, and ordering equipment and supplies. Optometrists who operate franchise optical stores also may have some of these duties.

Optometry programs include classroom and laboratory study of health and visual sciences, as well as clinical training in the diagnosis and treatment of eye disorders. Courses in pharmacology, *optics*, vision science, biochemistry, and systemic disease are included.

Business ability, self-discipline, and the ability to deal tactfully with patients are essential for success. The work of optometrists requires attention to detail and manual dexterity.

Optometrists wishing to teach or conduct research may study for a master's or Ph.D. degree in visual science, physiological optics, neurophysiology, public health, health administration, health information and communication, or health education. One-year postgraduate clinical residency programs are available for optometrists who wish to obtain advanced clinical competence. Specialty areas for residency programs include family practice optometry, pediatric optometry, geriatric optometry, vision therapy and rehabilitation, low-vision rehabilitation, cornea and contact lenses, refractive and ocular surgery, primary eye care optometry, and *ocular* disease.

Chapter 2
Anatomy and Physiology of the Eye

INTRODUCTION
ANATOMY OF THE EYE
  ▶ Eyeball
  ▶ Visual Pathway
  ▶ Ocular Appendages
PHYSIOLOGY OF THE EYE
  ▶ Eyelid
  ▶ Tears and Tear Film
  ▶ Cornea
  ▶ Sclera
  ▶ Aqueous Humor
  ▶ Lens
  ▶ Vitreous Body
  ▶ Retina

2.1 INTRODUCTION

The eye is a visual organ, which consists of two eyeballs and their surrounding *appendages*, *visual pathways* and *visual centers* which assist eyeball movement and protect it. Light emitted by different objects in space cause different visual cells in *retina* to excite and produce vision. The most suitable *electromagnetic wave* to cause human visual response is 400~700 nm. The eyeball is mainly composed of two parts, refractive conduction system and photosensitive imaging system. Refractive system includes *cornea*, *lens* and *vitreous body*. Photosensitive imaging system refers to retina. *Optic nerve* and *optic pathway* transmit the nerve impulse produced by retina to the visual center, and complete visual behavior through cerebral cortex integration.

2.2 ANATOMY OF THE EYE

Eye *anatomy* mainly studies the structure of normal eyes, revealing the *morphology*, structural characteristics and association with surrounding *tissues* and organs of human eyes. This section will be introduced according to three parts: eyeball, visual pathway and *ocular* appendages.

2.2.1 Eyeball

Eyeball is divided into two parts: eye wall and eye content. The eye wall is divided into three layers: the outer layer is composed of cornea and *sclera*, the middle layer is composed of *iris*, *ciliary body* and *choroid*, and the inner layer is retina. The inner structures are lens, *aqueous humor* and vitreous body (*Figure 2-1*).

2.2.1.1 Cornea

Cornea is the anterior 1/6th of the fibrous coat, located at the front end of the eye. It is *transparent*, *avascular*, *elastic* and has a large diopter. The surface is covered with *tear film*. The membrane is round and oval when viewed from the front due to the *asymmetry* of conjunctival and scleral coverage, but still round when viewed from the back. Around the cornea is the *limbus*, which is connected with the sclera, just like a watch case embedded in the dial. In the neonatal stage, the *corneal diameter* is about 9~10 mm, and the corneal diameter of children over 3 years old is close to that of adults. The average transverse diameter of cornea in adult male is about 11~12 mm, and the longitudinal diameter is about 10~11 mm, which is slightly smaller in female than in male. If the diameter is less than 10 mm, it is called *pathological* small cornea, and if it is greater than 13 mm, it is called pathological large cornea. The circular area of the central *pupil* region of the cornea, which is about 4 mm in diameter, is approximately spherical, and the radius of *curvature* of each point is basically equal, while the middle area and edge outside the central area are relatively flat, and the radius of curvature of each point is not equal. The radius of curvature measured from the anterior cornea is 7.8 mm in horizontal direction, 7.7 mm in vertical direction and 6.22~6.80 mm in posterior surface.

Corneal thickness varies with site, age and pathological state. Under normal circumstances, the central part is the thinnest, averaging about 0.5 mm, and the peripheral part is the thickest, averaging about 1 mm. Corneal thickness tends to become thinner with age. So, children are thicker than adults and adults are thicker than the elderly. Cornea is divided into five layers from front to back, which are *epithelial cell layer*, *anterior elastic layer*, *stroma layer*, *posterior elastic layer* and *endothelial cell layer* (*Figure 2-2*). Cornea is an avascular tissue, which is simple in composition but very regular in arrangement, thus ensuring its good light transmittance and refraction.

Limbus is the transitional area among cornea, conjunctiva and sclera. The limbus structure is different from cornea. There is no elastic layer, the stroma layer gradually loses transparency, and it is rich in capillaries, lymphatic vessels, fibroblasts and so on. Especially the outer 2/3 of it can be seen radially arranged papilla-like processes, which are palisade-like, called Vogt grid. Studies have confirmed that some cells in Vogt grid are limbal stem cells. Limbal stem cells play an important role in maintaining corneal epithelial regeneration (*Figure 2-3*).

2.2.1.2 Sclera

Sclera constitutes the posterior 5/6 of the outer fibrous membrane of the eye, which is mainly composed of *collagen fibers*. Outside of the sclera is the fascia sac of the eye, and the lacuna between them is the suprascleral cavity. The inner surface is close to the choroid, and the potential gap between them is the suprachoroidal space. Bleeding or *exudation* during trauma or *inflammation* can accumulate in this gap. The thickness of sclera varies with location and age. The posterior sclera is the thickest, about 1 mm, and gradually thins from the equator to the equator, which is about 0.4~0.6 mm. The muscle attachment point is the thinnest, about 0.3 mm, and about 0.6 mm from the equator to the limbus. Generally, sclera is white, but children are blue-white because sclera is thinner than adults so the part of the color of choroid can be seen, while the elderly are yellowish-white because of fat deposition.

Although the sclera is spherical, it is not completely spherical. The anterior scleral is connected with the cornea. A shallow sulcus can be seen inside and outside the junction of corneoscleral margin, which is called external scleral sulcus and internal scleral sulcus. The internal scleral sulcus is where scleral venous sinus and *anterior chamber* angle are located, and the posterior edge of the internal scleral sulcus bulges to form scleral process, which is the attachment of ciliary muscle. The posterior scleral foramen is the passage through which the optic nerve passes. Here, the inner 1/3 sclera and choroid together form the cribriform plate, and the outer 2/3 evolves into dura mater. It can be seen that the cribriform plate is a weak place at the back of the eye. At the same time, the scleral expansion ability at the cribriform plate is limited. When the optic nerve edema, it will cause optic nerve crush *injury* or even *atrophy*. In addition, there are many foramens to ensure the nerves and blood vessels passing through the sclera, such as vortex veins, pass about 4 mm behind the scleral equator.

2.2.1.3 Iris

Iris is part of the uveal tissue located in front, which is a disc-shaped pigmented septum with a small round hole in the center, named pupil. The iris *periphery* is attached to the anterior edge of ciliary body, which is called *iris root*, and extends to the center to the front of lens, dividing the space between lens and cornea into *anterior chamber* and *posterior chamber*. The size of pupil can vary with the intensity of light, and the pupil diameter is about 2.5~4 mm in normal circumstances. The color of iris is related to the amount of *pigment* contained in iris.

The anterior surface of the iris forms many uneven folds due to the radial arrangement of blood vessels in the parenchyma, which are called *iris texture* and *recess*. About 2 mm near the pupil edge, there is a circular serrated bulge line, which is called *iris curling wheel*, also known as *iris small ring*. Iris curling wheel divides the anterior surface of iris into central pupil area and peripheral ciliary area. The iris is thickest at the iris ring, thinning inward to the pupil edge, and thinning outward to the iris root, so it is easy to break the iris root when eye contusion occurs. Irregularly sized pits can be seen near the iris ring, which are called *iris pits* or *Fuchs recesses*. There are many radial bulges in ciliary area, which is the path of iris blood vessels. The back of the pupil edge of the iris is closely attached to the lens and supported by lens. When the lens is abnormal or removed, the iris may tremor due to the loss of support.

2.2.1.4 Ciliary body

The ciliary body is located in the middle of uvea, which is an annular tissue and with the width of 6~7 mm. The front edge is connected with the root of iris, and the membrane junction is serrated, which is called *ora serrata* (*Figure 2-4*). The fine section of the ciliary body is slightly triangular, with the top extending backward to the serrated edge, the base pointing to iris, and the anterolateral angle attached to scleritis. The ciliary body consists of a thicker ciliary crown (*Pars plicata*) in the front 1/3 and a thin and flat part in the back 2/3. The width of ciliary crown is about 2 mm, with abundant blood vessels. There are 70 ~ 80 longitudinal ridges with different sizes on the inner surface, named *ciliary processes,* which can greatly increase the surface area of aqueous humor secreting cells. In the space between ciliary processes, there are fibers of lens *suspensory ligament* attached to the surface of ciliary crown. The surface of the part extending backward from the ciliary crown to the front of the serrated edge is smooth and flat, and the width of the pars plana is about 4 mm.

On the outer surface of the eye, the anterior boundary of the ciliary body is 1.5 mm posterior to the limbus, and the ciliary crown is 2~3 mm posterior to the limbus, the flat part is 3.5 ~ 6.0 mm posterior to the limbus, the nasal side is slightly anterior, and the temporal side is slightly posterior. Pars plana is an important anatomical structure with few blood vessels. Vitrectomy incision from here can avoid bleeding and damage to lens and retina. Therefore, it is very important to be familiar with the anatomical location of ciliary body for posterior segment surgery.

2.2.1.5 Choroid

Choroid is the posterior part of uvea, which is a brown-black vascular structure rich in pigment. It is located between sclera and retina, with the anterior boundary starting from serrated edge and posterior part ending around *optic disc*. The thickness varies greatly with the filling degree of blood vessels, because the choroid is mainly composed of blood vessels. The inner surface of choroid is closely connected with the pigment epithelium of retina by Bruch's membrane, and there is a potential lacuna between the outer surface and sclera, called *suprachoroidal cavity*, which is connected with the brown-black layer of sclera by means of this cavity. The ciliary long and short arteries and ciliary long and short nerves all pass through this lacuna. Choroid is the most abundant blood vessel tissue in eye, which provides blood for the outer retina and *macular* area.

2.2.1.6 Retina

Retina is the innermost layer of eye wall. It is a membrane composed of nerve tissue, which extends forward and covers the ciliary body and the posterior surface of the iris. The posterior boundary is around the optic nerve papilla, the outer side is connected with Bruch membrane of choroid, and the inner side is surrounded by vitreous body. The retina is a hyaline membrane, which is red in vivo due to the influence of blood flow and rhodopsin in *rod* cells. The retina near the optic disc is thicker, about 0.56 mm, the retina at the serrated edge is thinner, only 0.1 mm, and the retina at the *fovea* is thinnest. The retina is tightly attached in two places. One is around the optic disc, and the other is the serrated edge. Retina can be divided into two parts: sensory part and non-sensory part. The retina extending forward from the optic nerve to the serrated edge can feel the stimulation of light, which is called the receptive part, also called the retinal visual part. The retina extending forward from the serrated edge and covering the ciliary body and the posterior surface of the iris does not contain nerve tissue and cannot feel the stimulation of light, so it is called the non-receptive part, also called the blind part of retina (*Figure 2-5*).

There is a discoid structure with a diameter of about 1.5 mm and a clear boundary about 3.0 mm on the nasal side of the posterior pole of the eye, which is called *optic disc* or *optic papilla*. It is the place where retinal nerve fibers gather and pass through the eye wall, and it is also the place where the central retinal artery and vein enter and exit. The optic disc is round or vertically oval in shape, with a vertical diameter slightly larger than the horizontal diameter and pale pink. In the center located a small concave with slightly lighter color called *optic cup* or *physiologic excavation*. Dark gray dots are faintly visible in optic cup, which is called *scleral sieve foramen*. There are individual differences in the position, shape, size and depth of the cup. The optic cup/disc (C/D) of normal people is mostly below 0.3. The size of optic cup in normal eyes is related to the area of optic disc, that is, the larger the optic disc, the larger the optic cup. There are a large number of optic nerve fibers passing through the optic disc, but there are no optic cells, so there is no ability to feel light stimulation, which is called "physiological blind spot". Central retinal arteries and veins, which are divided into four branches: superior nasal, inferior nasal, superior temporal and inferior temporal, all pass though the center of optic disc and distribute in retina to supply nutrition to the inner layer of retina.

Located at the posterior pole of retina, about 3 mm on the temporal side of optic disc, there is an oval shallow depression with a diameter of about 5 mm, which is light yellow in color and is called *macula lutea*. In the center of the macula is a small concave, called *fovea centralis*, which is located slightly lower than 3.5~4 mm outside the temporal edge of the optic disc. The visual acuity in fovea centralis is the best. During *ophthalmoscope* examination, it can be seen a reflection point the size of a needle tip in the fovea, which is called fovea reflex. There is no retinal blood vessel distribution in macula, and it is highly transparent. The retina here is extremely thin, and there are only cone cells at the bottom of fovea, with the highest density. Each cell is conducted one-to-one with the connected *bipolar cells* and *ganglion cells*, so fovea is the place with the sharpest vision and the strongest ability to distinguish colors (*Figure 2-6*).

2.2.1.7 Aqueous humor, anterior chamber, posterior chamber

The anterior chamber is a space between cornea, iris and lens, which is filled with aqueous humor. Its anterior boundary is the back of cornea and a small part of sclera, and its posterior boundary is the anterior surface of iris, a part of ciliary body and the anterior surface of lens in pupil area. The anterior chamber is filled with aqueous humor with a volume of 0.2 ml. The central depth of the anterior chamber is about 2.5~3 mm, which gradually becomes shallower to the periphery. The anterior chamber is deeper in *myopia* and shallower in *hyperopia*.

The peripheral part of the anterior chamber is a recess formed by the back of the limbus and the front of the iris root, which is called the *angle of anterior chamber*. The anterolateral side of the angle of anterior chamber is the corneal limbus, and the medial of the posterior side is the root of iris and the front end of ciliary body. The two parts migrate each other to form the angle of anterior chamber, which is slightly blunt and round, so it is not a true geometric angle. The *trabecular meshwork* and *scleral sinus (Schlemm canal)* are contained in the scleral sulcus at the posterior part of the anterolateral wall of the anterior chamber angle, which is an important channel for aqueous humor drainage and is closely related to the occurrence of *glaucoma* (*Figure 2-7*).

The posterior chamber is an annular cavity between the posterior iris, the front end of ciliary body, the front of lens suspensory ligament and the front of lens, with a volume of about 0.06 ml. The posterior chamber is filled with aqueous humor, which communicates with the anterior chamber through pupils.

Aqueous humor is a colorless and transparent liquid that fills the anterior chamber and posterior chamber of eye. Its main function is to maintain *intraocular pressure* and provide nutrition for cornea, lens and vitreous body. At the same time, it also plays a role in supporting eye wall and *refraction*.

2.2.1.8 Lens

Lens is an elastic biconvex transparent body, which is suspended between iris and vitreous body by the suspension ligament of lens. The front of the lens is slightly in contact with the pupil margin, and the back is located in the lens fossa in front of the vitreous body. The lens can be divided into front and back sides, the edge where the two sides meet is called *equator*, the vertices of the front and back surfaces are called anterior and posterior poles respectively, and the connecting lines of the front and posterior poles form the lens *axis*. The distance between equatorial part of lens and ciliary process is 0.5 mm. The curvature of the anterior and posterior surfaces of the lens is different. The radius of curvature of the anterior surface is about 9~10 mm, and that of the posterior surface is about 5.5~6 mm. The size, especially the thickness of the lens increases slowly with age. In the static state, the diameter of the adult lens is about 9~10 mm and the thickness is about 4~5 mm. When the lens changes pathologically, the size also changes. For example, the lens volume can increase significantly during the dilatation period of senile cataract, but the lens can become significantly thinner during the over-maturity period.

2.2.1.9 Vitreous

Vitreous is a colorless and transparent *gel*, which accounts for about 4/5 of the posterior volume of the eye. It is located behind the lens, and other parts are attached to the retina and ciliary body. There is a disk-shaped depression on the posterior surface of the vitreous body facing the lens, which is used to accommodate the lens, called vitreous depression, and there is a potential gap between them, called posterior lens space.

Vitreous body consists of vitreous cortex, central vitreous body and central canal. The peripheral part of vitreous body is thick, which is called vitreous cortex, while the interior of vitreous body is thin, which is called central vitreous body. The surface tissue of cortex is thick, forming the limiting membrane, which is not the real vitreous membrane. There are few cells in vitreous, and most of them are distributed on the cortical surface.

2.2.2 Visual Pathway

Visual pathway refers to all the pathways of visual nerve impulse conduction from retina to visual center of occipital lobe of brain. It includes optic nerve, optic chiasma, optic tract, lateral geniculate body, optic radiations and visual cortex (*Figure 2-8*).

2.2.2.1 Optic nerve

The *optic nerve* refers to the segment from the papilla of optic nerve to the optic chiasma, with a total length of about 42~50 mm. It is divided into four sections according to its location.

- *Intrabulbar segment*: The nerve fibers of retina are assembled into a bundle, which starts from optic nerve papilla and goes backward to pass through scleral lamina cribrosa, with a length of about 1.0 mm.
- *Intraorbital segment*: From posterior scleral foramen to optic foramen, it is the longest segment of optic nerve, about 25~30 mm, slightly S-shaped curved, which is beneficial to the rotation of eyeball.
- *Intraductal segment*: It is a segment of optic nerve passing through optic canal, which is about 6~10 mm. The diameter of the bone canal is small, so it is easy to cause obvious nerve compression due to fracture or lesion of the bone canal, resulting in visual impairment.
- *Intracranial segment*: It is a segment between the posterior foramen of optic canal and the forefoot of optic chiasma, which is about 10 mm.

2.2.2.2 Optic chiasma

Optic chiasma is the place where the optic nerves on both sides of the anterior and upper sella turcica meet, where the fibers from the nose cross with the fibers from the contralateral nose when crossing the midline, and the fibers from the temporal half of retina enter the ipsilateral optic bundle through the lateral side of optic chiasma. Because of the characteristics of nerve fibers running in optic chiasma, the visual field damage is different when there are lesions in different parts of optic chiasma.

2.2.2.3 Optic tract

Optic tract is a nerve bundle from optic chiasma to lateral geniculate body. Each optic tract is composed of nerve fibers from the temporal side of ipsilateral retina and the nasal side of contralateral retina, that is, fibers from the right half of both eyes constitute the right optic bundle, and fibers from the left half of both eyes constitute the left optic bundle.

2.2.2.4 Lateral geniculate body

The *lateral geniculate body* belongs to a part of diencephalon and has a saddle-shaped shape. Optic nerve fibers enter the lateral geniculate body. After replacing neurons here, new fibers are emitted to form visual radiation.

2.2.2.5 Optic radiations

Optic radiations originate from the lateral geniculate body and end in the occipital visual cortex of the brain. This section is the longest section in the visual path. The visual cortex is located in the striatum area on the medial side of the occipital lobe of the brain. *Brodmann 17*, the striatum where the visual center is located, is the projection area of visual radiation fibers, and each occipital striatum receives the projection of temporal fibers in the ipsilateral eye and nasal fibers in the contralateral eye. In addition, the parastatal area (*Brodmann 18*) close to the striatum and the peristriatal area (*Brodmann 19*) around the striatum do not directly receive visual fiber projection, but play a very important role in the perception and integration of visual information and the joint movement of both eyes.

2.2.2.6 Light reflex

When external light irradiates into the eye through the pupil, it causes pupil reflex to shrink, which is called *pupil light reflex*. The eyes irradiated by light have pupil contraction, which is called *direct reflection of light*. The contralateral eye that is not illuminated also has *miosis*, which is called *indirect reflection of light*. The afferent fibers of the light reflex pathway walk with the visual fibers, pass through the optic nerve and optic chiasma, then divided into crossed and non-crossed fibers along with the visual fibers to join the bilateral optic bundles. When approaching the lateral geniculate body, the light reflex fibers leave the optic bundles and stop at the anterior tectal nucleus. After replacing the neurons in this nucleus, the emitting fibers terminate in the ipsilateral and contralateral Edingger-Westphal nucleus (*E-W nucleus*). Then efferent fibers emit from bilateral E-W nuclei, join oculomotor nerve into orbit, exchange neurons in sleeping ganglion, and distribute to pupil sphincter through short ciliary nerve. When one optic nerve is completely injured, the direct light reflex of the eye disappears, but the indirect light reflex still exists. If one optic bundle is damaged, the direct light reflection of the pupil ligament on the hemianopia side of both eyes disappears, but the indirect light reflection exists (*Figure 2-9*).

2.2.2.7 Near reflex

Near reflex is the three reflexes that appear simultaneously when both eyes look at near objects, including pupil *contraction*, binocular convergence and ciliary muscle contraction. After the transmission impulse reaches the visual cortex through the visual pathway, the visual cortex is connected with the eye movement center of frontal lobe, from which the fibers descend through the oculomotor nucleus and the ventral nucleus of oculomotor nerve, and then enter the orbit together with the oculomotor nerve. After the ciliary ganglion exchanges neurons, the postganglionic fibers innervate the pupil *sphincter muscle* and ciliary muscle of both eyes to complete the pupil contraction and ciliary muscle contraction reflex. At the same time, the *oculomotor nerve* innervates the medial rectus muscles of both eyes, causing them to contract and complete the collective.

2.2.3 Ocular Appendages
2.2.3.1 Eyelids

Eyelids are located in front of the eye, which can protect the eye from trauma, strong light, smoke, foreign bodies, etc. Changes in the size of eyelid fissure caused by eyelid contraction can help pupils adjust the light entering the eye.

The eyelid is divided into upper eyelid and lower eyelid. The upper eyelid is bounded by eyebrows, while the lower eyelid continues with the surrounding skin without obvious boundary. Some people have a transverse sulcus near the eyelid edge on the upper eyelid surface, which is called the upper eyelid sulcus, which is caused by the traction of the subcutaneous tissue attached to the eyelid by the levator muscle fiber. This sulcus is the most obvious when the eyelid fissure is enlarged, that is, the double eyelid. The lower eyelid sulcus is not as obvious as the upper eyelid. The free edge of eyelid is called *lid margin*, and the fissure between upper and lower eyelid margin is called *palpebral fissure*, which is the entrance of conjunctival sac. The junction of the upper and lower eyelid margins is called *medial canthus* and *lateral canthus* respectively. The distance between the inner and outer canthus is called the length of eyelid fissure, which is about 27~28 mm in adults. When the eye opens naturally and looks straight ahead, the upper eyelid covers 2~3 mm below the upper edge of cornea, while the lower eyelid is tangent to the lower edge of cornea. The distance between the midpoints of the upper and lower eyelid margins is called the height of eyelid fissure, and the average is 8 mm in adults. The outer canthus angle is acute, with an included angle of about 30°~ 40°, and can be 60° when eyes are extremely opened. The inner canthus is slightly blunt and round, not directly in contact with the eye, and there is a small triangular gap between it and the eyeball, which is a tear lake. There is an oval red bulge called *lacrimal caruncle*, and there is a reddish crescent fold called *plica semilunaris* outside the lacrimal caruncle. The semilunaris is degenerated tissue, which is equivalent to the third eyelid of lower animals and can allow the eye to move fully outward (*Figure 2-10*).

The width of the upper and lower eyelid edges is about 2 mm, and the surface is smooth.

Each eyelid edge is divided into front and back lips, and the front lip is blunt and round, with eyelid skin as the boundary, from which 2 ~ 3 lines of eyelashes are born. The posterior lip is sharp, bounded by eyelid conjunctiva, at right angles to conjunctiva and in contact with eye surface, and there is an opening of *meibomian gland* in front of the posterior lip. There is a gray and thin line between the anterior and posterior lips, called gray line. During operation, the eyelid fold can be split into anterior and posterior parts along the gray line. The anterior part includes skin, subcutaneous tissue and *orbicularis muscle*, and the posterior part includes *tarsal plate* and conjunctiva. There is a small bulge at the inner canthus of the upper and lower eyelid margin, which is called lacrimal *papilla*, and there is a small hole in the center of lacrimal papilla, which is the opening of *lacrimal canaliculus*. Tears in conjunctival sac are guided from *lacrimal puncta* to lacrimal canaliculus and finally discharged into nasal cavity. Born from the front lip of the upper and lower eyelid margin, it is the short hair with thick rod, which has the function of shielding dust and light. The eyelashes of the upper eyelid are about 100~150, arranged in 2~3 rows, and bent 10° ~130° forward and upward. The eyelashes of the lower eyelid are slightly shorter, and bent 100° ~110° forward and downward. Therefore, when closing the eyelid, the eyelashes of the upper and lower lid are not interlaced, and the nerve endings of eyelash hair follicles are rich, which are very sensitive to touch and can cause *blink reflex*. Eyelashes can be continuously updated, and after being pulled out, they can generally reach the original length in about 10 weeks.

2.2.3.2 Conjunctiva

Conjunctiva is a thin and transparent mucous membrane, which covers the inner surface of eyelid and the front surface of eyeball, thus connecting eyelid and eyeball. The anterior part of the conjunctiva opens in the fissure of the eyelid and forms a sac-like space with the cornea as the base, which is called *conjunctival sac*. The depth of conjunctival sac is different at different positions, and the deepest is in the upper part and temporal side. All conjunctiva are continuous with each other and can be divided into three parts according to their different positions: *palpebral conjunctiva* covers the inner surface of eyelid, *bulbar conjunctiva* covers the anterior surface of eyeball, and *fornical conjunctiva* is the transitional part between them.

2.2.3.3 Lacrimal apparatus

Lacrimal apparatus can be divided into secretory part and excretory part. The secretion part includes lacrimal gland and accessory lacrimal gland, and the excretion part includes lacrimal puncta, lacrimal canaliculus, common lacrimal duct, *lacrimal sac* and *nasolacrimal duct*. Besides, conjunctival sac, lacrimal caruncle, semilunar fold, orbicularis muscle and eyelid margin also play an important role in tear excretion (*Figure 2-11*).

2.2.3.4 Extraocular muscles

There are six *extraocular muscles*, including four rectus muscles and two oblique muscles, which are *superior rectus muscle*, *inferior rectus muscle*, *lateral rectus muscle*, *medial rectus muscle*, *superior oblique muscle* and *inferior oblique muscle*. Except the inferior oblique muscle, the other five extraocular muscles and *levator palpebrae muscle* all originate from the common tendinous ring (also known as *Zinn ring*) or closely connected with it (*Figure 2-12*).

- *Superior rectus muscle*: The superior rectus muscle starts from the upper part of the common tendinous ring, runs forward and outward under the levator palpebrae superioris muscle, forms an angle of 23 with the visual axis, crosses the upper direction of the superior oblique tendon near the equator of the eyeball, enters the ocular fascia, and attaches to the sclera at 7.7 mm behind the limbus. The tendon is 5.8 mm, and the nasal end of the attachment line is slightly forward than the pre-side. The superior rectus muscle is innervated by oculomotor nerve and supplied by the external muscular branch of ophthalmic artery and the branch of lacrimal artery. The main function of the superior rectus muscle is to make the eye rotate up and rotate inward.

- *Inferior rectus muscle*: The inferior rectus muscle runs from the lower part of the common tendinous ring and below the optic foramen along the orbital floor. The inferior rectus muscle is innervated by oculomotor nerve and supplied by the internal muscular branch of ophthalmic artery and the branch of infraorbital artery. The main function of the inferior rectus muscle is to make the eyeball rotate downward, inward and outward.

- *Lateral rectus muscle*: The lateral rectus muscle originates from the outer upper part of the common tendinous ring, and a small part originates from the orbital surface of the great wing of sphenoid bone. Along the lateral orbital wall, the tendon is attached to the sclera at 6.9 mm behind the limbus, and the tendon is 8.8 mm. The abducent nerve enters the lateral rectus muscle from the medial side at 15 mm from the muscle origin and innervates the muscle. The lateral rectus muscle is supplied by the lateral muscular branch of ophthalmic artery and the branch of lacrimal gland artery. Its function is to make the eye turn outward simply.

- *Medial rectus muscle*: The medial rectus muscle is the largest muscle in the extraocular muscles, which originates from the lower part of the common tendinous ring, the inner and lower part of the optic foramen at the orbital apex, runs forward along the medial orbital wall, and attaches to the sclera at 5.5 mm behind the limbus, with a tendon length of 3.7 mm. The medial rectus muscle is also innervated by oculomotor nerve, and the nerve branch enters the muscle from the middle and posterior 1/3 of the lateral side of the muscle. The medial rectus muscle is supplied by the internal muscular branch of ophthalmic artery. The function is to make the eye turn inward.

- *Superior oblique muscle*: The superior oblique muscle is the thinnest, longest, most complicated and therefore most vulnerable extraocular muscle, which originates from the bone surface above the optic foramen and is closely connected with the common tendinous ring. The trochlear nerve enters from above the muscle where

it originated and innervates the muscle. The superior oblique muscle is supplied by the external muscle branch of the service artery. The main function is to make the eyeball rotate inward, downward and outward.
- *Inferior oblique muscle*: The inferior oblique muscle is the only extraocular muscle that starts in front of the orbit. It starts at the orbital surface of the maxilla outside the lacrimal sac fossa, and a few muscle fibers start from the lacrimal fascia covering the lacrimal sac. The muscles and tendons are short, innervated by oculomotor nerve, and the nerve branches enter from the upper part of the middle of the muscle. The muscle is supplied by the internal muscle branch of ophthalmic artery and the branch of infraorbital artery. Its main function is to make the eye rotate outward, up and outward.

2.3 PHYSIOLOGY OF THE EYE

2.3.1 Eyelid

Eyelid is the *physiological* barriers to protect eyes. Eyelashes arranged neatly at the edge of eyelid can prevent foreign bodies from the human eye and act as stress instantaneous receptors. The blood circulation of eyelid is abundant, and the wound heals rapidly after trauma, but the tissue reaction is strong after pathogenic microorganism *infection*, so the focus is easy to spread. Blink is the most common regular or stressful action of eyelid closing and opening in turn. The physiological functions include: avoiding foreign bodies and trauma, evenly coating tear film on eye surface, helping tear circulation and cleaning cornea, etc. Blink can be divided into two types: autonomous blink and non-autonomous blink. Autonomic blinking is a blink whose frequency and degree are controlled by subjective consciousness. Then, the involuntary blink can be divided into spontaneous blink and reflective blink. Spontaneous blink is a regular blink spontaneously produced without any external stimulation. The main physiological function of spontaneous blink is to reform and redistribute tears in front of cornea, while reflex blink is a defensive blink reaction to some external stimuli. It can be visual stimulation or tactile stimulation, such as sudden strong light and unexpected contact with eye surface, eyelashes, eyelid skin and eyebrows, which can cause reflective blinking.

2.3.2 Tears and Tear Film

Tears have the functions of keeping the eye surface moist, clean, nourishing and protecting the eye surface tissues. The continuous and normal *secretion* of tear quality and quantity depends on the normal tissues and organs producing tears and the normal drainage ways of tears. Tear film is formed by uniformly coating tears on the eye surface. Tear film consists of three parts from outside to inside, which are *lipid layer*, *aqueous layer* and *mucous layer* in turn. Most of tears are water, secreted by main lacrimal gland and accessory lacrimal gland, living in the middle layer of tear film. Lipid layer is secreted by *meibomian gland*, insoluble in water, and its main components are cholesterol and wax, which can prevent water loss and maintain tear film morphology. The inner mucus layer is attached to corneal *epithelium*. It is mainly secreted by ocular surface epithelial cells (including non-goblet cells and conjunctival goblet cells), and its main components are protein, hexosamine, etc. Its function is to strengthen the hydrophilicity of corneal epithelial cells and increase the ocular surface adhesion of tear film. Basal tears were mainly secreted by Krause's accessory lacrimal glands (67%) and Wolfring's accessory lacrimal glands (33%). The secretion volume was 1.0~1.2 μl/min, and the total amount of tears in 24 hours was 10 ml. Normal tear film rupture occurs every 15~40 seconds, which is called *tear film rupture time*. The tear film repaired and updated by blinking, 10~12 times per minute. Its main functions are to clean conjunctival sac, moisten eye surface, resist infection, transport oxygen, glucose, white blood cells, etc. Besides, it also takes away horn conjunctival metabolites and inflammatory substances. When stimulated by boundary, such as foreign bodies, physical and chemical *toxic* substances, etc., it can cause reflex lacrimal glands to secrete a large amount of tear, which can be used to clean ocular surface tissues and dilute toxic substances. At this time, the total amount of tears secreted can reach 10 times of the basic tear amount, and the tears contain *lysozyme* and other substances.

2.3.3 Cornea

The main physiological functions of cornea are: maintaining the integrity of eye and protecting the contents of eye, transmitting light and participating in refraction, and sensing environment and external stimuli.

- *Maintaining the integrity of the eye and protecting the contents of the eye*: Cornea and sclera together form the outer wall of the eyeball to bear the intraocular pressure, and play an important role in maintaining the shape of the eyeball. Cornea is mainly composed of *collagen fibers*, so it has certain elasticity and toughness, and has resistance to intraocular pressure and external forces. This resistance depends on the thickness of cornea and the neatness of collagen fibers. The decrease of corneal thickness or the formation of *corneal scar* will definitely reduce the resistance of cornea to internal and external pressure. At present, *corneal refractive surgeries* are very popular. But the surgeries also reduce corneal resistance to varying degrees. For example, excimer *laser* surgery makes the thickness of the center of cornea thinner, thus increasing the ability of cornea to expand under the action of external force. In this way, the measurement result will be low when measuring intraocular pressure, especially when using indentation *tonometer*, the low intraocular pressure will be more obvious. Radial keratotomy will greatly reduce the resistance of cornea to the outside world, and may cause eye rupture under the action of slight external force. Usually, corneal thickness is affected by corneal epithelium, corneal endothelium function, exposure and other factors. Corneal epithelium is the second biological barrier of eyes (tears are the first biological barrier). The corneal epithelial cells are connected tightly, and the old and the new are constantly replaced. The corneal epithelium is renewed once every 5~7 days, which can resist the invasion of chemistry and *microorganisms* to a certain extent. Corneal endothelium is the barrier between horn and leg stroma and aqueous humor, and the pump function of corneal endothelium keeps cornea in a certain *hydration* state.

- *Transmittance*: An important feature of cornea is transparency, that is, allowing light to pass through, which is the basis of eye visual function. The permissible light length of normal cornea is 365~2500 nm, and the permeability of different rays is different. About 80% of 400 nm rays can pass through the cornea, while 100% of 500~1200 nm rays can pass through the cornea. In addition, corneal transparency also depends on the normal structure and function of tear film, corneal epithelium, corneal stroma and corneal endothelium, and the constant water content of corneal stroma.
- *Participating in the optical system*: The cornea is the most refractive tissue in the optical system of the eye. The *refractive index* of cornea is 1.377, the *refractive power* of anterior surface is 48.8 D, the refractive power of posterior surface is −5.8 D, and the total refractive power is 43 D, accounting for 70% of the total refractive power. It can be seen that corneal luminosity has great potential for change, which is also the basis of many refractive operations on cornea at present.
- *Osmosis*: There is no blood vessel in cornea. Nutrients and metabolites enter and leave cornea through osmosis, which not only has important physiological significance, but also is very important for local drug treatment of eyes. Corneal epithelium and endothelial cells are closely connected, and the cell surface is rich in lipids, so nonpolar substances are easy to pass through, while stroma is easy to pass through water-soluble *polar* substances. Therefore, bidirectional substances are easy to enter the anterior chamber through cornea. When corneal lesions occur, corneal *permeability* will be enhanced.
- *Perception of environment and external stimuli*: Cornea is the most sensitive area of human, with abundant nerve endings, which can sensitively feel external *stimuli*, and is of great significance for the body to feel external adverse stimuli and respond quickly. There are three kinds of corneal *perception*: cold, pain and touch.

2.3.4 Sclera

The physiological functions of sclera mainly include:
- Forming the external barrier of eye content together with cornea and conjunctiva;
- Avoiding light;
- Being attachment point of extraocular muscles.

The sclera bears the outward pressure of the eye content all time, so the sclera has certain elasticity and toughness. When the intraocular pressure rises, the sclera can expand within a certain range and enhance its resistance to intraocular pressure. When the intraocular pressure is low, the increase of a certain amount of eye content will cause a small increase in intraocular pressure, but when the intraocular pressure is high, the same increase in eye content will cause a large increase in intraocular pressure. This characteristic of sclera is called scleral rigidity or distensibility. Understanding this is helpful to understand the influence of scleral hardness on intraocular pressure measurement. Compared with the flat tonometer, the indentation tonometer causes great changes in ocular volume, so scleral hardness has a greater influence on the measurement results of indentation tonometer. For example, in high myopia, the eye wall is thin, the sclera is easy to expand, and the intraocular pressure measured by indentation tonometer will be low. The second important function of sclera is to form a "black box". Compared with cornea, sclera is *opaque*, which ensures that light only enters human eyes through refractive system for imaging. Another important function is that all extraocular muscles are attached to the scleral. When the attachment point of muscles is changed, the position and movement direction of eye can be changed.

2.3.5 Aqueous Humor

Aqueous humor is produced by ciliary process epithelium of ciliary body, which fills posterior chamber and anterior chamber, with a total amount of 0.15~0.3 ml, and its main component is water. Aqueous humor comes from *plasma*, but it is different from plasma. The protein content in aqueous humor is about 0.2 mg/ml, which is only 1/400~1/300 of its plasma content. The *albumin* content in aqueous humor is relatively higher than that in plasma, while the *globulin* content is relatively lower than that in plasma. When the *blood-aqueous humor barrier* is destroyed due to trauma and other reasons, the protein content in aqueous humor increases sharply, and the aqueous humor flashes in clinical *slit lamp examination*. The pH value of aqueous humor is 7.3~7.5, the specific gravity is 1.003, the viscosity is 1.025~1.100, and the refractive index is 1.336. Aqueous humor is in dynamic circulation, which is produced by ciliary process epithelium of ciliary body, reaches posterior chamber, enters anterior chamber through pupil, then enters Schlemm tube through trabecular meshwork from the angle amber, and finally enters anterior ciliary vein on sclera surface and returns to blood circulation. This outflow pathway is pressure-dependent. In addition, a small part of aqueous humor is drained from uveoscleral route (about 10% ~ 20%) or absorbed through iris surface recess (trace). If any part of the aqueous humor circulation channel is blocked, it will lead to an increase in intraocular pressure.

2.3.6 Lens

Lens is a simple epithelial cell structure, without blood vessels and nerve tissue, and its nutrition comes from aqueous humor and vitreous body. In normal eyes, the lens is equivalent to a convex lens of 20 D, which is one of the most important refractive media. The *zonule* fibers of lens are connected with ciliary body, and the contraction and relaxation of ciliary muscle drive the thickness of the whole lens to become thinner or thicker through zonule fibers, thus changing its tortuous force. In addition, the lens can absorb *ultraviolet rays* and protect the retina. With the increasing of age, the weight of lens gradually increases, the nucleus of lens becomes larger and larger, the elasticity gradually decreases and the transparency gradually decreases too.

2.3.7 Vitreous Body

The vitreous body consists of 98% water and 2% collagen and hyaluronic acid. Vitreous body is a component of refractive medium of eyes, which has three physical characteristics: viscoelasticity, permeability and transparency. The vitreous body can support, damp and nourish the surrounding tissues such as lens and retina.

2.3.8 Retina

As a transparent film, the main function of retina is to feel light and transmit visual information to the center through optic nerve, and form vision through the integration and processing of the center. The cone and rod cells of retina capture photons and convert them into electrical stimulation, which is called light conversion. This process is completed in the outer segment of photoreceptor-cone-rod cells. The nerve impulses of *photoreceptors* are transmitted to ganglion cells through bipolar cells. Then nerve fibers (axons) emitted by ganglion cells converge to the optic disc. The distribution of neurons in different positions of retina is different, so vision is divided into peripheral vision and central vision. For example, there are only cone cells in the central area of macula, and the closer it is to the center, the denser the neurons are, which makes it have the highest *visual sensitivity*. The vision perceived by the macular fovea is called central vision, and the vision perceived by the retina around the fovea is called peripheral vision. Central vision has a high degree of discrimination, including bright vision and color vision. Peripheral vision provides spatial positioning information. The peripheral retina can feel dark light better because of more rod cells. When the peripheral retina is damaged, night blindness will occur. The fibers in the macular area are bounded by horizontal sutures and arranged in an upper and lower arc shape to reach the temporal side of the optic disc. This fiber bundle is called the macular fiber bundle of the optic disc. The temporal peripheral fibers are also divided into upper and lower sides and enter the optic disc. The fibers in the upper and lower parts of the nasal retina converge directly to the optic disc.

In addition, the outermost layer of retina, namely retinal pigment epithelium, has the ability to absorb and scatter light, control the fluid and nutrients in subretinal space (function of blood-retinal barrier), regenerate and synthesis of visual pigment, synthesis of growth factors and other metabolites, maintain retinal attachment, pentosis and digestion of metabolic waste of photoreceptors, maintain electrical steady state, regeneration and repair after trauma and surgery and so on. Retinal pigment epithelium is very important to maintain the function of photoreceptors. It is also affected by many retinal and choroidal diseases. In fact, many clinical changes in retinal diseases occurred in the pigment epithelium, not in the retina, because the retina is transparent.

Chapter 3
Clinic Methods in Optometry

INTRODUCTION
CASE HISTORY
OPTOMETRIC EXAMINATION

- ► External Ocular Examination
- ► Testing of Visual Acuity
- ► Amplitude of Accommodation (AMP)
- ► Color Vision
- ► Cover Test
- ► Stereopsis
- ► Worth 4-Dot Test (W4D)
- ► Near Point of Convergence (NPC)
- ► Hirschberg Test
- ► Extraocular Motilities (EOM)
- ► Pupil Test
- ► Finger Counting Visual Fields Test

3.1 INTRODUCTION

The purpose of the clinical procedures for ocular examination is to provide students and practitioners with detailed step-by-step procedures. Clinically, our task is to understand the patient's chief complaint, and according to their clinical manifestations and signs to make a corresponding judgment, complete the relevant examinations, make a reasonable diagnosis, and give advice and treatment plan. In this chapter, we focus on the main points of the diagnostic process, including how to take case history, how to do entrance tests, how to summarize the findings of the examinations for the patients along with recommendations for appropriate care, referrals, and follow-up care.

3.2 CASE HISTORY

Clinically, the most important thing is to communicate with the patients. Good patient communication is conducive to the smooth progress of the examination process, improve the accuracy of diagnosis, improve patient compliance, reduce patient complaints, and make each clinician's and patient's experience more pleasant. Doctor-patient communication is a skill that can be learned and improved over time. Optometrists should establish a caring relationship with the patients, showing enough compassion, empathy, and respect for the patients. Optometrists also need to ask some questions about the patient's chief complaint, visual function, ocular and systemic health, risk factors, and lifestyle. In this way, we can make differential diagnosis easier, and do patient education better. Thus, a case history provides the doctor or clinician with a comprehensive background on a patient's medical or psychological condition.

- *Ocular history*

Have you ever been diagnosed with Refractive Error/Cataract/Glaucoma?

- *Medical history*

Are you allergic to any medicine?

Have you taken any medicine recently?

- *Review of systems*

Is there anything wrong with your Skin/Heart/Immune System?

Do you have any neurological problems?

- *Symptoms of common eye problems*

Do you have any Eye Pain/Eye Redness/Itchy Feeling/Blurry Vision?

When did your vision start to deteriorate?

Do you think these symptoms are affecting your life?

- *Family history*

Do you have any immediate family members with Diabetes/High Blood Pressure/High Cholesterol?

- *Social history*

Do you Drive/Smoke?

In this part, the only thing we can do is to know the patient's health, and the more we know, the more accurate the diagnosis will be.

3.3 OPTOMETRIC EXAMINATION

3.3.1 External Ocular Examination

Not only eye diseases, many systemic diseases have manifestations observable in the external ocular examination. To identify gross abnormalities of the eye and adnexa, in general, the examiner should look for anything odd or unusual about the patient and any asymmetries between one side of the body and the other, and pay particular attention to the face and eyes. The external eye structures include the eyelids and surrounding tissues, conjunctiva, lacrimal apparatus, cornea, anterior chamber, and so on.

Clinically, we usually use *slit lamp* to accomplish this operation. Slit lamp is a microscope with a bright light used during an eye exam. It gives ophthalmologists and optometrists a closer look at the different structures at the front of the eye and inside the eye. It's a key tool in determining the health of patient's eyes and detecting eye diseases. There are many lighting methods which can be used. The most commonly used way are *direct illumination method* and *diffusion illumination method*. Adjust the intensity to provide enough light for examination, but keep in mind that high intensity light will be uncomfortable for many patients especially if the pupils are dilated. A neutral density filter can also be used to reduce light intensity. Most slit lamps offer stepwise magnification between 6x and 40x. Lower power (6x~10x) maintains a wide field of view is optimal for general examination. High power can be used to examine the fine structure of pathologic features identified at low power.

For patients, there is no special preparation needed before the slit lamp exam. For clinicians, asking a patient to place his/her chin in the chin rest and his/her forehead against the forehead band. This keeps patient's head steady during the exam. Clinicians may use eye drops containing yellow dye to help visualize problems on the front surface of the eye. Dilating drops may also be used to widen patient's pupil for a better look at the back of the eye. Clinicians will sit down facing a patient and look through the microscope at his/her eyes. Clinicians will then turn on the slit lamp and focus a narrow, high-intensity beam of light towards patient's eye. Although the light is very bright, it will not cause any damage to the eye and should not cause any pain. Remember, before beginning your exam, ensure that the forehead band, chin rest, and handles have been thoroughly cleaned with alcohol.

3.3.2 Testing of Visual Acuity (VA)

Visual acuity is the ability of your eyes to distinguish between objects that you see when standing at a specific distance. It is also called visual sharpness, or clarity of vision. Visual acuity is the most common clinical measurement of visual function and measures the smallest size letters that can be reliably identified at a specified distance.

Eyecare professionals measure visual acuity by conducting various tests that designate how sharp or clear someone can see from 20 feet away. Visual acuity is the first thing eye doctors assess when examining a patient because it gives a baseline of the person's eyesight. VA is usually tested by reading an eye chart. Room illumination should maximize the contrast on the visual acuity chart used. (Higher illumination is needed for printed charts and dimmer illumination is needed for projected or computerized charts.) The Snellen eye chart, with its familiar rows of letters in decreasing sizes, is the most common visual acuity test.

When the examiner wants to measure the patient's visual acuity both with (cc) and without (sc) correction, the visual acuity should be measured without correction first. While standing or sitting 20 feet from the chart, patients are instructed to read each row until he/she no longer can. This measurement describes people's ability to see an object from 20 feet away compared to a person with normal vision. VA is usually written as a fraction. The upper number represents the distance you stood at when viewing the chart. The lower digit is the distance in which a person with normal vision would see the object you read well. For example, 20/25 vision means that you need to be 20 feet away to see clearly what a person with normal vision can see from 25 feet away. If a patient cannot see the largest object at 20 feet, instruct the patient to move closer to the chart, stop at the distance he/she can see the object clearly. If a patient reads the 6/6 line but gets 2 letters incorrect, you would record this as 6/6 (−2). If a patient gets more than 2 letters wrong, then the previous line should be recorded as visual acuity. When recording the visual acuity, it should state whether this vision was unaided (SC), with glasses(CC) or with a pinhole (PH).

If the patient cannot see the letters at any distance, initiate the following testing, stopping at the level at which the patient can accurately respond.

- *Counting fingers*
- *Hand motion*
- *Light projection*
- *Light perception*

Similarly, we can test the near visual acuity by using near eye charts. Pinhole visual acuity is also important. Pinhole occluder consists of multiple, small apertures amidst a dark background. The pinhole occluder works along the same basis as pupil constriction in bright conditions causing an improvement in visual acuity. Through a smaller pupil, the effects of minor ocular irregularities—such as refractive error or paracentral cornea or lens opacities—are diminished. The examiner should determine if a decrease in vision is correctable by glasses. Viewing the far acuity chart through a pinhole will increase the patient's depth of focus and decrease the retinal blur. If the retina and visual pathway are free of abnormalities, the patient's acuity will improve. (Pinhole visual acuity test should be taken if the VA is worse than 20/30 at both distant and near through the habitual or prescribed correction.) Using pinhole visual acuity can offer the clinician a great deal of important information. It functions as a rapid tool to screen for best-corrected visual acuity without having to employ refractive techniques. It also suggests that if a pinhole fails to improve vision, the reduced vision is likely a result of pathology, whether a structural defect or functional change. Additionally, it is a readily available and cost-effective alternative to determine postoperative visual endpoints for patients undergoing cataract surgery.

3.3.3 Amplitude of Accommodation (AMP)

AMP means the difference between the refractive power of the eye when adjusted for vision at the far point and when adjusted for vision at the near point. This procedure measures a patient's ability to change the focus of the eye's lens in response to close stimulation. The results are indicated by diopter. There are 2 methods widely used:

3.3.3.1 Method 1 Push-up method and pull-away method

This test subjectively measures the AMP under monocular conditions. Test the right eye first, and then the left eye, instruct the patient to look at the one or two lines larger than his/her near visual acuity.

①*Push-up method*: Instruct the patient to keep the target clear, and slowly move the target towards the patient. Ask the patient to report when he/she sees the target become and remain blurry, measure the distance between the target and patient's spectacle plane in centimeters, and convert the linear distance into diopters (D1). For example, if the distance is 8 cm, D1=1/0.08=12.5 D.

②*Pull-away method*: Hold the target very close to the patient. The patient would see it blurry. Slowly move away the target and ask the patient to report when he/she sees it become clear. Measure the distance between the target and patient's spectacle plane in centimeters, and convert the linear distance into diopters (D2). For example, if the distance is 10 cm, D1=1/0.10=10 D.

In this test, it is critical to accurately measure the distance, because even small errors in measurement can lead to large differences in results. To reduce this problem, this test can be measured through −4.00 DS lenses. This modification moves the endpoint further away from the patient and allows more exact measurement of the endpoint. Finally, AMP=0.5×(D1+D2). It is best to repeat the measurement three times and then take the average. After we get the result, we need to judge whether the patient's AMP is abnormal through Hofstetter's formulas: The average amplitude at any age = 18.5−1/3 age. The minimum amplitude expected for a given age = 15−1/4 age.

3.3.3.2 Method 2 Minus lenses method

This test subjectively measures the amplitude of accommodation under monocular conditions. Test the right eye first, then the left eye, and instruct the patient to look at a vertical line of letters or a block of letters of about 20/30 at 40 cm. Instruct the patient to keep the letters clear, slowly add minus lenses until the patient reports he can't keep it clear, and record the endpoint (when the first sustained blur appears). The amount of minus added during the test plus 2.50 D (the accommodative demand for a near point card at 40 cm) is the total amplitude of accommodation. The expected value for minus lens amplitude is about 2 D less than that for the push-up method.

3.3.4 Color Vision

The sun, lasers and light bulbs all generate light waves. Humans perceive a small part of the spectrum known as visible light. Other parts of the spectrum include infrared and ultraviolet light, which human eyes cannot perceive. Light rays travel from a light source to objects and surfaces in the environment. Some light is absorbed and some is reflected.

When these reflected waves reach the human eye, the human brain converts them into color perception. Color vision is one of the brain's greatest inventions. The human visual system will tell you that an apple is red and a pear is yellow. The colors are actually all in your head, and, of course, in your eyes. Therefore, color perception is the result of a complex interplay between the light, the eyes and the brain.

However, there are some people who have trouble perceiving colors, which may indicate a disease or a deficiency in the visual system, such as so-called color blindness. The term "color blindness" isn't exactly accurate, because people with this condition still have eyesight, and they may also see some colors. If a person has color blindness, it means he/she see colors differently than most people. Most of the time, color blindness makes it hard to tell the difference between certain colors. The most common type of color blindness makes it hard to tell the difference between red and green. Another type makes it hard to tell the difference between blue and yellow. Only a small percentage of people affected by color blindness have a complete lack of color perception. That's why medical science prefers the term "color vision deficiency". Usually, color blindness runs in families. Color vision is particularly significant for the evaluation of macular cone cells and optic nerve function, also can be used to screen for acquired or hereditary color vision defects.

There are several ways to choose from, such as the Ishihara test, FM-100 test, and Panel D-15 test. In China, Yu's color blindness test has been widely used in the national recruitment of students, workers, and conscripts. There's no cure for color blindness, but special glasses and contact lenses can help it. Most color-blindness patients are able to adapt and have no problems with everyday activities.

3.3.5 Cover Test

Assessing binocular function is an important aspect of the comprehensive eye examination. Binocular vision is a visual efficiency skill where both eyes work together in a precise and coordinated way. Good binocular vision provides sustained, single, and comfortable vision, which is the basis of depth perception. The cover test is a measurement of eye posture (or eye alignment). This test is used to evaluate and quantify ocular deviations that may be present, which are called tropias and phorias (*Figure 3-1*). A tropia is a physical misalignment in one or both eyes that can also be called strabismus. On the other hand, a phoria is a deviation that may only be present when the eyes are not looking at the same object. One key difference: whether fusion is maintained or not. To test for the different types of deviations and quantify their magnitude, the cover test is divided into two main parts: *cover-uncover test* and *alternating cover test*. Both parts of the evaluation are performed at distance and near. It is to be performed while the patient wears any applicable habitual correction. Instruct the patient to look at the target and keep it clear. The target for both distance and near test should be a single letter, one or two lines above the patient's best corrected visual acuity of the worse eye. The near target should be held approximately 40 cm away from the patient and control the patient's accommodation.

3.3.5.1 Cover-uncover test/Unilateral cover test(UCT)

The cover-uncover test differentiates between a phoria and a tropia and determines if a tropia is alternating or unilateral.

1) During the cover part

When both eyes are open, the clinician covers an eye with a hand or paddle for a few seconds and looks for the movement of the fellow eye to see if it moves to pick up fixation. Repeat it 2~3 times to verify your observation.

- If the patient has a phoria, each visual axis will be aligned with the target.
- If the patient has a tropia, one visual axis will be aligned with the target and the other visual axis will be misaligned with the target.

2) During the uncover part

When both eyes are open, the cover paddle is then removed, and the clinician looks for movement of the previously covered eye. We can differentiate alternating tropias from unilateral tropias (constant right or constant left tropias).

- A patient with an alternating tropia is able to keep either the right or left visual axis aligned with the target.
- A patient with a unilateral tropia habitually fixates with one eye and only fixates with the troping eye when the fixating eye is occluded. In esotropia, this adjustment is from medial to lateral; in exotropia, it is from lateral to medial.

3.3.5.2 Alternating cover test(ACT)

The alternating cover test does not differentiate between a phoria and a tropia, but determines the direction and magnitude of deviations. In this test, we have to keep one of the eyes covered all the time to keep fusion disrupted. For example, cover the right eye for 3 seconds, and then switch to cover the left eye, then back and forth several times. Remember waiting 3 seconds in between movements to allow time for the eyes to re-find your test target. We use the direction of movement of the eye to identify the direction of the deviation (*Table 3-1*). For example, if we see the patient's eye move from nasal to temporal, it shows the movement is "Out", so the direction of deviation is "Eso". Quantifying the angle using prism is necessary, but the angle may change with fatigue.

Table 3-1 The way to determine the direction of deviation

The Direction of Eye Movement as Eye Is Uncovered	Direction of Deviation
In	Exo
Out	Eso
Up	Hypo
Down	Hyper

3.3.6 Stereopsis

There are three grades of binocular vision: macular perception, fusion, stereopsis. Stereopsis is absent at birth and develops in children between 3 and 6 months of age. From infancy to old age, any interference in the process of perceiving depth can lead to defective stereopsis. For example, children with congenital cataracts cannot develop simultaneous perception if they are not corrected early enough. Another possibility is a child with anisometropia, which can lead to anisometric amblyopia, then the child cannot fuse the images from both eyes but rather produces two separate images in the brain. Because of the difference in visual acuity, the brain prefers to suppress the eye which has greater refractive error, which disrupt the stereopsis.

The purpose of stereopsis test is to measure the patient's depth perception. There are many test cards to choose from, such as Random Dot 2, Titmus, Bernell, TNO test, Random Dot E, and PASS (*Figure 3-2*). Clinically, we suggest using the Random Dot test which has fewer monocular clues. Before the stereopsis test, we need to give the patients near correction, polaroid glasses, or red-green glasses depending on the test used. Stereopsis is quantified by a unit known as seconds of arc. The expected findings of stereopsis at near is 20 seconds of arc.

3.3.7 Worth 4-Dot Test (W4D)

The Worth 4-Dot test is composed of four lights arranged in a diamond shape with a red light at the top, two green lights at the left and right sides, and a white light at the bottom (*Figure 3-3*). The Worth 4-Dot test is a simple tool for assessing suppression and fusion, which refers to test whether a person is using both eyes at the same time to see the object. Patients are instructed to wear red-green goggles and appropriate distance correction in place. The transmission characteristics of the red-green goggles are such that the eye wearing the red filter (usually the right eye) blocks green light to see only the top and bottom light. Another eye (usually the left eye wears green filter) can only see the two green lights and the bottom light. In this test, we should perform it twice (at distance and near). Actually, it is not necessary to ask about the color of the lights. The number of lights is seen with the right eye, left eye, and both eyes are more important.

During the test, we need to ask the patient some questions:
- Cover the patient's left eye and ask, "How many lights do you see?"
- Now cover the right eye and ask, "How many lights do you see?"
- Now with both eyes open ask, "How many lights do you see?"
- Now with both eyes open ask, "What color are they?"
- Now with both eyes open ask, "Where are they located?"
- Now with both eyes open ask, "Do all the lights appear at the same time, or do they flash on and off?"

There are four possible responses:

① "4 dots seen": When a patient sees all four dots, one is suspected of having either a normal binocular fusional response with no manifest strabismus or a harmonious anomalous retinal correspondence.

If retinal images differ in size due to aniseikonia or in clarity as in amblyopia, anisometropia that is not corrected, or unilateral eye diseases, it could be that the images of the two eyes are not fused because one eye is suppressed.

② "3 dots seen": If the patient only sees three green dots, it means he/she is only using his/her left eye and suppressing his/her right eye.

③ "2 dots seen": If the patient only sees two red dots, it means he/she is only using his/her right eye and suppressing his/her left eye.

④ "5 dots seen": If the patient has double vision, he/she will report that he/she sees five dots. Then ask the patient if the green dots are located to the right, left, above, or below the red dots.

- If the red dots are to the right of the green dots, the patient has an Eso deviation (uncrossed diplopia).
- If the red dots are to the left of the green dots, the patient has an Exo deviation (crossed diplopia).
- If the red dots are above the green dots, the patient has a left hyper deviation.
- If the red dots are below the green dots, the patient has a right hyper deviation.

TIPS:

① If suppression or diplopia is detected, turn off the room lights and repeat the test.

② In patients who show suppression, it's useful to repeat the test with the red-green goggles reversed to ensure an accurate assessment.

③ Determine which eye is suppressing then ask a patient to cover the eye that is not suppressing and to report whether or not the suppressed dots reappear. If the dots reappear, the patient has a suppression scotoma that only occurs in binocular vision. If the dots do not reappear, the patient has a unilateral scotoma.

④ If the central scotoma is suspected, ask the patient to continue fixating four dots and to report if the number of dots drops to either 3 or 2 at any time, slowly move the near target away from the patient and ask him to report when suppression occurs. If the patient sees all four dots at 3 metres, the test stops and record it "no suppression to 3 metres".

3.3.8 Near Point of Convergence(NPC)

We need to determine the patient's ability to converge the eyes while maintaining fusion. It is easy to perform and does not require any special equipment. Examiners only need a fixation target and a ruler. The results of the test should be noted with near point of convergence(NPC) and convergence recovery point(CRP). The normal NPC is about 6~10 cm and the CRP is about 15 cm. If the NPC is more than 10 cm, this is a sign of poor convergence.

The patient should sit in a comfortable chair and look directly at the fixation object, which is held in the mid-sagittal plane of the patient's head, approximately 50 cm from it. The room should be well illuminated so the examiner can notice changes in eye movements.

1) Method 1: Measured by penlight, used for initial screening

Move the target toward and away from the patient's eyes, get the break point and recovery point (in cm). Perform the test 5 times to see if there is any change. Usually, normal people will not show fatigue when the test is repeated.

① Break point: The examiner will move the fixation object slowly and smoothly in the mid-sagittal plane closer to the patient's nose. Moving speed should be proximately 40 cm in 10 seconds. Remember, explain to the patient that the object can become blurry, but he/she still needs to continue to fixate on it. Ask the patient to let you know when he/she sees the fixation object in double or until you see the patients' one eye lose fixation on the target.

② Recovery point: Move the target away from the patient's eyes, ask the patient to let you know when he/she sees the fixation object in single or until you see the patient's deviated eye regains fixation.

2) Method 2: Measured by penlight with red-green goggles, or accommodative targets only

These modified methods are used when you suspect the patient has convergence insufficiency(CI). In normal patients, the results should be the same in each method. If there is an obvious difference between the methods, the patient may have convergence insufficiency.

3.3.9 Hirschberg Test
3.3.9.1 Monocular test

Let the patient take off glasses, place the penlight toward the patient's eyes about 50~100 cm, and ask the patient to look at the light. Occlude the patient's left eye to test the right eye, and determine the location of the corneal light reflex to the pupil. Then occlude the patient's right eye to test the left eye. There are three possibilities:

- The corneal light reflex is in the center of the pupil.
- The corneal light reflex is slightly nasal to the center of the pupil $(+\lambda)$.
- The corneal light reflex is slightly temporal to the center of the pupil $(-\lambda)$.

3.3.9.2 Binocular test

This method can be used to determine the strabismus roughly, because the visual axes of both eyes under binocular conditions will be manifested. Similarly, let the patient take off glasses, place the penlight toward the patient's eyes about 50~100 cm, and ask the patient to look at the light binocularly. Determine the location of the corneal light reflexes in each eye with both eyes open, and compare them with the positions tested under monocular condition.

- If the corneal light reflexes are in the same location between monocular and binocular condition, it means no strabismus exists.
- If the corneal light reflexes are not in the same location between monocular and

binocular conditions, it means strabismus exists (*Table 3-2*).

Table 3-2 Relationship between the position of the corneal reflex
and the type of deviation on the Hirschberg test

Position of Corneal Reflex Relative to Position of Angle Lambda in the Fixating Eye	Type of Deviation
Nasal	Exo
Temporal	Eso
Above	Hypo
Below	Hyper

- The size of strabismus can be estimated by the location of the corneal light reflex, 1 mm of deviation of the reflex is equal to 22Δ (*Figure 3-4*).

3.3.10 Extraocular Motilities(EOM)

At first, we all know that the purpose of the extraocular muscles is to control the movement of globe. There are 6 extraocular muscles, superior rectus muscle(SR), inferior rectus muscle(IR), superior oblique muscle(SO), inferior oblique muscle(IO), lateral rectus muscle(LR), and medial rectus muscle(MR). The action of muscles is affected by globe position in the ocular orbit and muscle orientations.

The purpose of extraocular motility test is to investigate the integrity of the extraocular muscles and their nerves, to assess the patient's ability to perform version eye movements, and to determine if strabismus is comitant. When deviation of the visual axes remains constant in all fields of gaze, there is comitancy. When deviation of the visual axes changes with field of gaze, there is noncomitancy.

EOM test is also part of confrontational tests. The most common test for extraocular motility is the broad H test, which is a pursuit test done binocularly with penlight at a test distance of 30~40 cm. Broad H test tests the fields of action of the 6 extraocular muscles. Field of action means direction where a particular muscle has the greatest action. Having the patient without glasses, hold the penlight approximately 30~40 cm in front of the patient's eyes and ask the patient to follow the light source with their eyes rather than their head. Start at the primary position, then eight more (*Figure 3-5*). During the test, take care to ask the patient if they see the light source becoming double, or if they feel discomfort, pain, tension, etc.

There are three points that clinicians need to observe:
- The smoothness of movement.
- The accuracy of patient's eye following the penlight.
- The extent of movement.

If the patient reports any diplopia or double vision during the test, examiners need to do further tests, such as the muscle field with red lens, ductions procedures, and saccades procedures. If the patient does not report diplopia or double vision, and you see the patient follow the light smoothly to all positions of gazes binocularly, record it as SAFE or FESA.

3.3.11 Pupil Test

The physiology behind a "normal" pupillary reaction is a balance between the sympathetic and parasympathetic nervous systems (*Figure 3-6*). Sympathetic innervation leads to pupillary dilation. Parasympathetic innervation leads to pupillary constriction. Clinicians can assess the afferent and efferent neurological pathways through the pupil test.

There are 5 aspects of pupillary reaction which need to be assessed.

3.3.11.1 Appearance of pupil

There are 5 key features of a pupil.

① Size: Normal pupil size is about 2~8 mm, abnormally small (maybe caused by pilocarpine) or abnormally large (maybe caused by dilating drops or CN3 palsy) pupil should be concerned.

② Shape: Maybe round/circular, tadpole, irregular, festooned.

③ Position: Make sure the pupil is in the center of the eye.

④ Color: Normal pupil shows greyish black (may show grey, white or brown in a patient with cataract).

⑤ Symmetry: Normal condition should be less than 1 mm difference between two eyes.

3.3.11.2 Direct pupil response

Set the environmental illumination to dim, instruct the patient to look at the far target, then use the penlight or transilluminator shine to one eye, and observe the size of pupil and the speed of pupillary constriction. Likewise, test the other eye. Repeat the procedures.

3.3.11.3 Consensual pupil response

Set the environmental illumination to dim, instruct the patient to look at the far target, then use the penlight or transilluminator shine to the right eye, and observe the size of pupil and the speed of pupillary constriction in the left eye. Likewise, use the penlight or transilluminator to shine to the left eye, and observe the size of pupil and the speed of pupillary constriction in the right eye. Repeat the procedures.

3.3.11.4 Swinging flash light test

Set the environmental illumination to dim, instruct the patient to look at the far target, then move the light between two eyes quickly, leaving it on each eye for about 3 to 5 seconds, and compare the direct response of the right eye to the direct response of the left eye during this period(focusing on the size of pupil, dilation, and constriction). Repeat the procedures.

3.3.11.5 Accommodative(Near) response of the pupil

If one or two pupils fail to respond directly or consensually, or if their responses are sluggish, test the near response of the pupil. Instruct the patient to direct his/her gaze from the far target to the near target, in which looking for pupillary constriction. Then instruct the patient to direct his gaze toward the near target to the far target, in which looking for pupillary dilation.

At last, if all the pupillary functions are normal, record it as "PERRLA no APD" (*Figure 3-7*).

3.3.12 Finger Counting Visual Fields Test

Visual field test looks for visual field defects and their location. Central and peripheral vision is tested by using visual field tests. Careful detection of visual field defects can be diagnostic of many ocular and/or neurological conditions, including glaucoma or retinitis pigmentosa. In glaucoma, as well as other conditions, it is vital to repeat visual field test to track any changes over time. Examining visual fields is an integral part of a full ophthalmic evaluation. Several methods for assessing visual field loss are available, and the choice of which to use depends on the patient's age, health, visual acuity, ability to concentrate, and socio-economic status. Available techniques can test the full field (including confrontation, tangent screen, Goldmann perimetry and automated perimetry), or assess just the central field of vision, such as the Amsler Grid.

The purpose of finger counting visual fields test is to roughly screen for visual field defects. This technique is generally effective only for obvious visual field losses. At first, we need an overhead lamp and an occluder. Instruct the patient to remove his/her glasses. The examiner faces the patient at eye level, keeping the distance about 60~80 cm to patients. Instruct the patient to occlude his/her left eye and keep looking at your left eye with his/her right eye at all times. Tell the patient that you are going to show your fingers in his/her side vision, let him/her tell you how many fingers you are holding up. Place your hand in a plane midway between you and the patient. Your hand should be in the far periphery, but at a location where you will be able to distinguish the number of fingers exposed. Finger counting visual fields test is actually a form of visual acuity of the peripheral visual field. During the test, the patient's visual field is compared to your field, which is presumed to be full. Repeat the steps in the appropriate eight locations in the field, on each side of the four visual field meridian. Repeat the steps on the patient's left eye. Throughout the test, monitor the patient's fixation and keep reminding him/her to maintain fixation on your open eye. Record the results for each eye separately. If the patient's visual field is normal, record it as "Full". If the patient's visual field is abnormal, record it as "Restricted" followed by the location of the restriction. The expected findings are right eye full and left eye full.

Chapter 4
Refractive Error

EMMETROPIA

HYPERMETROPIA
- ▶ Etiology
- ▶ Clinical Types
- ▶ Nomenclature (Components of Hypermetropia)
- ▶ Symptoms
- ▶ Complications
- ▶ Treatment
- ▶ Aphakia
- ▶ Pseudophakia

MYOPIA
- ▶ Etiological Classification
- ▶ Clinical Varieties of Myopia
- ▶ Treatment of Myopia

ASTIGMATISM
- ▶ Regular Astigmatism
- ▶ Irregular Astigmatism

ANISOMETROPIA
- ▶ Etiology
- ▶ Clinical Types
- ▶ Status of Binocular Vision in Anisometropia
- ▶ Diagnosis
- ▶ Treatment

ANISEIKONIA
- ▶ Etiological Types
- ▶ Clinical Types
- ▶ Symptoms
- ▶ Treatment

4.1 EMMETROPIA

Emmetropia (optically normal eye) can be defined as a state of refraction, where in the parallel rays of light coming from infinity are focused at the sensitive layer of retina with the *accommodation* being at rest.

At birth, the eyeball is relatively short, having +2 to +3 hypermetropia. This is gradually reduced until by the age of 5~7 years the eye is *emmetropic* and remains so till the age of about 50 years. After this, there is tendency to develop hypermetropia again, which gradually increases until at the extreme of life the eye has the same +2 to +3 with which it started. This senile hypermetropia is due to changes in the crystalline lens. *Ametropia* (a condition of refractive error), is defined as a state of refraction, when the parallel rays of light coming from infinity (with accommodation at rest), are focused either in front or behind the sensitive layer of retina, in one or both the meridians. The ametropia includes myopia, hypermetropia and astigmatism. The related conditions *aphakia* and *pseudophakia* are also discussed here.

4.2 HYPERMETROPIA

Hypermetropia (hyperopia) or long-sightedness is the refractive state of the eye wherein parallel rays of light coming from infinity are focused behind the retina with accommodation being at rest. Thus, the posterior focal point is behind the retina, which therefore receives a blurred image.

4.2.1 Etiology

Hypermetropia may be axial, curvatural, index, positional and due to absence of lens.

① *Axial hypermetropia* is by far the commonest form. In this condition the total refractive power of eye is normal but there is an axial shortening of eyeball. About 1 mm shortening of the anteroposterior diameter of the eye results in 3 dioptres of hypermetropia.

② *Curvatural hypermetropia* is the condition in which the curvature of cornea, lens or both is flatter than the normal, resulting in a decrease in the refractive power of eye. About 1 mm increase in radius of curvature results in 6 dioptres of hypermetropia.

③ *Index hypermetropia* occurs due to decrease in refractive index of the lens in old age. It may also occur in *diabetics* under treatment.

④ *Positional hypermetropia* results from posteriorly placed crystalline lens.

⑤ Absence of crystalline lens either congenitally or acquired (following surgical removal or posterior dislocation) leads to aphakia —a condition of high hypermetropia.

4.2.2 Clinical Types

There are three clinical types of hypermetropia.

① *Simple or developmental hypermetropia* is the commonest form. It results from normal biological variations in the development of eyeball. It includes axial and curvatural hypermetropia.

② *Pathological hypermetropia* results due to either congenital or acquired conditions of the eyeball which are outside the normal biological variations of the development. It includes:
- Index hypermetropia (due to acquired cortical sclerosis).
- Positional hypermetropia (due to posterior subluxation of lens).
- Aphakia (congenital or acquired absence of lens).
- Consecutive hypermetropia (due to surgically over-corrected myopia).

③ Functional hypermetropia results from paralysis of accommodation as seen in patients with third nerve paralysis and internal ophthalmoplegia.

4.2.3 Nomenclature (Components of Hypermetropia)

Nomenclature for various components of the hypermetropia is as follows:

Total hypermetropia is the total amount of refractive error, which is estimated after complete *cycloplegia* with atropine. It consists of latent and manifest hypermetropia.

① *Latent hypermetropia* implies the amount of hypermetropia (about 1 D) which is normally corrected by the inherent tone of ciliary muscle. The degree of latent hypermetropia is high in children and gradually decreases with age. The latent hypermetropia is disclosed when refraction is carried after abolishing the tone with atropine.

② *Manifest hypermetropia* is the remaining portion of total hypermetropia, which is not corrected by the ciliary tone. It consists of two components, the facultative and the absolute hypermetropia.
- *Facultative hypermetropia* constitutes that part which can be corrected by the patient's accommodative effort.
- *Absolute hypermetropia* is the residual part of manifest hypermetropia which cannot be corrected by the patient's accommodative efforts.

Thus, briefly: Total hypermetropia = latent hypermetropia + manifest hypermetropia (facultative hypermetropia + absolute hypermetropia).

4.2.4 Symptoms

In patients with hypermetropia the *symptoms* vary depending upon the age of patient and the degree of refractive error. These can be grouped as under:
- *Asymptomatic.* A small amount of refractive error in young patients is usually corrected by mild accommodative effort without producing any symptom.
- *Asthenopic symptoms.* At times the hypermetropia is fully corrected (thus vision is normal) but due to sustained accommodative efforts patient develops asthenopic symptoms. These include tiredness of eyes, frontal or fronto-temporal headache, watering and mild *photophobia*. These asthenopic symptoms are especially associated with near work and increase towards evening.

- *Defective vision with asthenopic symptoms*. When the amount of hypermetropia is such that it is not fully corrected by the voluntary accommodative efforts, then the patients complain of defective vision which is more for near than distance and is associated with asthenopic symptoms due to sustained accommodative efforts.
- *Defective vision only*. When the amount of hypermetropia is very high, the patients usually do not accommodate (especially adults) and there occurs marked defective vision for near and distance.

The signs are:
- Size of eyeball may appear small as a whole.
- Cornea may be slightly smaller than the normal.
- Anterior chamber is comparatively shallow.
- *Fundus examination* reveals a small optic disc which may look more vascular with ill-defined margins and even may simulate *papillitis* (though there is no swelling of the disc, and so it is called pseudopapillitis). The retina as a whole may shine due to greater brilliance of light reflections (shot silk appearance).
- A-scan ultrasonography (biometry) may reveal a short antero-posterior length of the eyeball.

4.2.5 Complications

If hypermetropia is not corrected for a long time the following *complications* may occur:
- Recurrent styes, blepharitis or chalazia may occur, probably due to infection introduced by repeated rubbing of the eyes, which is often done to get relief from fatigue and tiredness.
- Accommodative convergent squint may develop in children (usually by the age of 2~3 years) due to excessive use of accommodation.
- *Amblyopia* may develop in some cases. It may be *anisometropic* (in unilateral hypermetropia), *strabismic* (in children developing accommodative squint) or *ametropic* (seen in children with uncorrected bilateral high hypermetropia).
- Predisposition to develop primary narrow angle glaucoma. The eye in hypermetropes is small with a comparatively shallow anterior chamber. Due to regular increase in the size of the lens with increasing age, these eyes become prone to an attack of narrow angle glaucoma. This point should be kept in mind while instilling *mydriatics* in elderly hypermetropes.

4.2.6 Treatment

Optical treatment. Basic principle of treatment is to prescribe *convex* (plus) lenses, so that the light rays are brought to focus on the retina. Fundamental rules for prescribing glasses in hypermetropia include:
- Total amount of hypermetropia should always be discovered by performing

refraction under complete cycloplegia.
- The spherical correction given should be comfortably acceptable to the patient. However the astigmatism should be fully corrected.
- Gradually increase the spherical correction at months interval till the patient accepts manifest hypermetropia.
- In the presence of accommodative convergent squint, full correction should be given at the first sitting.
- If there is associated amblyopia, full correction with *occlusion therapy* should be started.

Modes of prescription of convex lenses:
- *Spectacles* are most comfortable, safe and easy method of correcting hypermetropia.
- *Contact lenses* are indicated in unilateral hypermetropia. For cosmetic reasons, contact lenses should be prescribed once the prescription has stabilised. Otherwise, they may have to be changed many times.
- *Surgical treatment* of hypermetropia.

4.2.7 Aphakia

Aphakia literally means absence of crystalline lens from the eye. However, from the optical point of view, it may be considered a condition in which the lens is absent from the pupillary area. Aphakia produces a high degree of hypermetropia.

4.2.7.1 Causes
- *Congenital* absence of lens. It is a rare condition.
- Surgical aphakia occurring after removal of lens is the commonest presentation.
- Aphakia due to absorption of lens matter is noticed rarely after trauma in children.
- Traumatic extrusion of lens from the eye also constitutes a rare cause of aphakia.
- Posterior dislocation of lens in vitreous causes optical aphakia.

4.2.7.2 Optics of aphakic eye
Following optical changes occur after removal of crystalline lens:
- Eye becomes highly hypermetropic.
- Total power of eye is reduced to about +44 D from +60 D.
- The anterior focal point becomes 23.2 mm in front of the cornea.
- The posterior focal point is about 31 mm behind the cornea, i.e. about 7 mm behind the eyeball. (The antero-posterior length of eyeball is about 24 mm.)
- There occurs total loss of accommodation.

4.2.7.3 Clinical features
Symptoms:
- Defective vision. Main symptom in aphakia is marked defective vision for both far and near due to high hypermetropia and absence of accommodation.
- Erythropsia and cynopsia, i.e. seeing red and blue images. This occurs due to

excessive entry of ultraviolet and infrared rays in the absence of crystalline lens.

Signs:
- Limbal scar may be seen in surgical aphakia.
- Anterior chamber is deeper than normal.
- Iridodonesis, i.e. tremulousness of iris can be demonstrated.
- Pupil is jet black in colour.
- Purkinje's image test shows only two images.
- Findus examination shows hypermetropic small disc.
- *Retinoscopy* reveals high hypermetropia.

4.2.7.4 Treatment

Optical principle is to correct the error by convex lenses of appropriate power so that the image is formed on the retina.

Modalities for correcting aphakia include spectacles, contact lens, intraocular lens, and refractive corneal surgery.

1) Spectacles

Spectacles prescription has been the most commonly employed method of correcting aphakia, especially in developing countries. Presently, use of aphakic spectacles is decreasing. Roughly, about +10 D with cylindrical lenses for surgically induce astigmatism are required to correct aphakia in previously emmetropic patients. However, exact number of glasses will differ in individual case and should be estimated by refraction. An addition of +3 to +4 D is required for near vision to compensate for loss of accommodation.

Advantages of spectacles: It is a cheap, easy and safe method of correcting aphakia.

Disadvantages of spectacles:
- Image is magnified by 30%, so not useful in unilateral aphakia (produce diplopia).
- Problem of spherical and chromatic aberrations of thick lenses.
- Field vision is limited.
- Prismatic effect of thick glasses.
- Roving ring Scotoma (Jack in the box phenomenon).
- Cosmetic blemish especially in young aphakia.

2) Contact lenses

Advantages of contact lenses over spectacles include:
- Less magnification of image.
- Elimination of *aberrations* and *prismatic* effect on thick glasses.
- Wider and better field of vision.
- Cosmetically more acceptable.
- Better suited for uniocular aphakia.

Disadvantages of contact lenses are:
- More cost.
- Cumbersome to wear, especially in old age and in childhood.

- Corneal complications may be associated.

3) Intraocular lens

Intraocular lens implantation is the best available method of correcting aphakia. Therefore, it is the commonest modality being employed nowadays.

4) Refractive corneal surgery

Refractive corneal surgery is under trial for correction of aphakia. It includes:
- Keratophakia. In this procedure, a lenticule prepared from the donor cornea is placed between the lamellae of patient's cornea.
- Epikeratophakia. In this procedure, the lenticule prepared from the donor cornea is stitched over the surface of cornea after removing the epithelium.
- Hyperopic Lasik.

4.2.8 Pseudophakia

The condition of aphakia when corrected with an intraocular lens implant (IOL) is referred to as pseudophakia or artephakia.

Refractive status of a pseudophakic eye depends upon the power of the IOL implanted as follows:
- Emmetropia is produced when the power of the IOL implanted is exact. It is the most ideal situation. Such patients need plus glasses for near vision only.
- Consecutive myopia occurs when the IOL implanted overcorrects the refraction of eye. Such patients require glasses to correct the myopia for distance vision and may or may not need glasses for near vision depending upon the degree of myopia.
- Consecutive hypermetropia develops when the under-power IOL is implanted. Such patients require plus glasses for distance vision and additional +2 to +3 D for near vision.

Note: Varying degree of surgically-induced astigmatism is also present in pseudophakia.

Signs of pseudophakia (with posterior chamber IOL):
- Surgical scar may be seen near the limbus.
- Anterior chamber is slightly deeper than normal.
- Mild iridodonesis (tremulousness) of iris may be demonstrated.
- Purkinje image test shows four images.
- Pupil is blackish in colour but when light is thrown in pupillary area shining reflexes are observed. When examined under magnification after dilating the pupil, the presence of IOL confirmed.
- Visual status and refraction will vary depending upon the power of IOL implanted as described above.

4.3 MYOPIA

Myopia is a type of refractive error in which parallel rays of light coming from infinity are focused in front of the retina when accommodation is at rest.

4.3.1 Etiological Classification
- *Axial myopia* results from increase in anteroposterior length of the eyeball. It is the commonest form.
- *Curvatural myopia* occurs due to increased curvature of the cornea, lens or both.
- *Positional myopia* is produced by anterior placement of crystalline lens in the eye.
- *Index myopia* results from increase in the refractive index of crystalline lens associated with nuclear sclerosis.
- Myopia due to excessive accommodation occurs in patients with *spasm* of accommodation.

4.3.2 Clinical Varieties of Myopia
4.3.2.1 Congenital myopia
Congenital myopia is present since birth. However, it is usually diagnosed by the age of 2~3 years. Most of the time the error is unilateral and manifests as anisometropia. Rarely, it may be bilateral. Usually the error is of about 8 D to 10 D which mostly remains constant. The child may develop convergent squint in order to preferentially see clear at its far point (which is about 10~12 cm). Congenital myopia may sometimes be associated with other congenital anomalies such as *cataract*, microphthalmous, aniridia, megalocornea and congenital separation of retina. Early correction of congenital myopia is desirable.

4.3.2.2 Simple myopia
Simple or *developmental myopia* is the commonest variety. It is considered as a physiological error not associated with any disease of the eye. Its prevalence increases from 2% at 5 years to 14% at 15 years of age. Since the sharpest rise occurs at school going age, i.e. between 8 years to 12 years, it is also called school myopia.

1) Etiology

It results from normal biological variation in the development of eye which may or may not be genetically determined. Some factors associated with simple myopia are as follows:
- Axial type of simple myopia may signify just physiological variation in the length of the eyeball or it may be associated with precocious neurological growth during childhood.
- Curvatural type of simple myopia is considered to be due to underdevelopment of the eyeball.
- Role of diet in early childhood has also been reported without any conclusive results.
- Role of *genetics*. Genetics plays some role in the biological variation of the

development of eye, as prevalence of myopia is more in children with both parents myopic (20%) than the children with one parent myopic (10%) and children with no parent myopic (5%).
- Theory of excessive near work in childhood was also put forward, but did not gain much importance. In fact, there is no truth in the folklore that myopia is aggravated by close work, watching television and by not using glasses.

2) Symptoms
- Poor vision for distance (short-sightedness) is the main symptom of myopia.
- Asthenopic symptoms may occur in patients with small degree of myopia.
- Half shutting of the eyes may be complained by parents of the child. The child does so to achieve the greater clarity of stenopaeic vision.

3) Signs
- *Prominent eyeballs*. The myopic eyes typically are large and somewhat prominent.
- Anterior chamber is slightly deeper than normal.
- Pupils are somewhat large and a bit sluggishly reacting.
- Fundus is normal, and rarely temporal myopic crescent may be seen.
- Magnitude of refractive error. Simple myopia usually occur between 5 and 10 years of age and it keeps on increasing till about 18~20 years of age at a rate of about −0.5 ± 0.30 D every year. In simple myopia, usually the error does not exceed 6 D to 8 D.

Diagnosis is confirmed by performing retinoscopy.

4.3.2.3 Pathological myopia

Pathological/degenerative/progressive myopia, as the name indicates, is a rapidly progressive error which starts in childhood at 5~10 years of age and results in high myopia during early adult life which is usually associated with degenerative changes in the eye.

1) Etiology

It is unequivocal that the pathological myopia results from a rapid axial growth of the eyeball which is outside the normal biological variations of development. To explain this spurt in axial growth various theories have been put forward. So far no satisfactory hypothesis has emerged to explain the etiology of pathological myopia. However, it is definitely linked with heredity and general growth process.
- *Role of heredity*. It is now confirmed that genetic factors play a major role in the etiology. As the progressive myopia is familial, more common in certain races like Chinese, Japanese, Arabs and Jews, but uncommon among Africans, Nubians and Sudanese. It is presumed that heredity-linked growth of retina is the determinant in the development of myopia. The sclera due to its distensibility follows the retinal growth but the choroid undergoes degeneration due to stretching, which in turn causes degeneration of retina.
- *Role of general growth process*. Lengthening of the posterior segment of the globe commences only during the period of active growth and probably ends with

the termination of the active growth. Therefore, the factors (such as nutritional deficiency, debilitating diseases, endocrine disturbances and indifferent general health) which affect the general growth process will also influence the progress of myopia.

2) Symptoms
- Defective vision. There is considerable failure in *visual function* as the error is usually high. Further, due to progressive degenerative changes, an uncorrectable loss of vision may occur.
- Muscae volitantes, i.e. floating black opacities in front of the eyes are also complained of by many patients. These occur due to degenerated liquified vitreous.
- *Night blindness* may be complained by very high myope having marked degenerative changes.

3) Signs
- Prominent eye balls. The eyes are often prominent, appearing elongated and even simulating an exophthalmos, especially in unilateral cases. The elongation of the eyeball mainly affects the posterior pole and surrounding area, the part of the eye anterior to the equator may be normal.
- Cornea is large.
- Anterior chamber is deep.
- Pupils are slightly large and react *sluggishly* to light.
- Fundus examination reveals the following characteristic signs: a. Optic disc appears large and pale and at its temporal edge a characteristic myopic crescent is present. Sometimes peripapillary crescent encircling the disc may be present, where the choroid and retina is distracted away from the disc margin. A super-traction crescent (where the retina is pulled over the disc margin) may be present on the nasal side. b. Degenerative changes in retina and choroid are common in progressive myopia. These are characterised by white atrophic patches at the macula with a little heaping up of pigment around them. Foster-Fuchs' spot (dark red circular patch due to sub-retinal *neovascularization* and choroidal *haemorrhage*) may be present at the macula. *Cystoid degeneration* may be seen at the periphery. In an advanced case there occurs total retinal atrophy, particularly in the central area. c. Posterior *staphyloma* due to ectasia of sclera at posterior pole may be apparent as an excavation with the vessels bending backward over its margins. d. Degenerative changes in vitreous include *liquefaction*, *vitreous opacities*, and posterior vitreous detachment (PVD) appearing as Weiss' reflex.
- Visual fields show contraction and in some case ring scotoma may be seen.
- ERG reveals subnormal electroetionogram due chorioretinal atrophy.

4) Complications
- Retinal detachment.

- Complicated cataract.
- Vitreous haemorrhage.
- Choroidal haemorrhage.
- Strabismus fixed convergence.

4.3.3 Treatment of Myopia

- Optical treatment of myopia constitutes prescription of appropriate *concave* lenses, so that clear image is formed on the retina. The basic rule of correcting myopia is converse of that in hypermetropia, i.e. the minimum acceptance providing maximum vision should be prescribed. In very high myopia undercorrection is always better to avoid the problem of near vision and that of minification of images. Modes of prescribing concave lenses are spectacles and contact lenses. Their advantages and disadvantages over each other are the same as described for hypermetropia. Contact lenses are particularly justified in cases of high myopia as they avoid peripheral distortion and minification produced by strong concave spectacle lens.
- Surgical treatment of myopia is becoming very popular nowadays.
- General measures empirically believed to effect the progress of myopia (unproven usefulness) include balanced diet rich in vitamins and proteins and early management of associated debilitating disease.
- Low vision aids (LVA) are indicated in patients of progressive myopia with advanced degenerative changes, where useful vision cannot be obtained with spectacles and contact lenses.
- Prophylaxis (genetic counselling). As the pathological myopia has a strong genetic basis, the hereditary transfer of disease may be decreased by advising against marriage between two individuals with progressive myopia. However, if they do marry, they should not produce children.

4.4 ASTIGMATISM

Astigmatism is a type of refractive error wherein the refraction varies in the different meridia. Consequently, the rays of light entering in the eye cannot converge to a point focus but form focal lines. Broadly, there are two types of astigmatism: regular and irregular.

4.4.1 Regular Astigmatism

The astigmatism is regular when the refractive power changes uniformly from one meridian to another (i.e. there are two principal meridia).

4.4.1.1 Etiology

- Corneal astigmatism is the result of abnormalities of curvature of cornea. It constitutes the most common cause of astigmatism.

- Lenticular astigmatism is rare. It may be: a. Curvatural due to abnormalities of curvature of lens as seen in lenticonus. b. Positional due to tilting or oblique placement of lens as seen in subluxation. c. Index astigmatism may occur rarely due to variable refractive index of lens in different meridia.
- Retinal astigmatism due to oblique placement of macula may also be seen occasionally.

4.4.1.2 Types of regular astigmatism

Depending upon the axis and the angle between the two principal meridia, *regular astigmatism* can be classified into the following types.

- *With-the-rule astigmatism.* In this type the two principal meridia are placed at right angles to one another but the *vertical* meridian is more curved than the *horizontal*. Thus, correction of this astigmatism will require the concave cylinders at 180° ± 20° or convex cylindrical lens at 90° ± 20°. This is called "with-the-rule" astigmatism.
- *Against-the-rule astigmatism* refers to an astigmatic condition in which the horizontal meridian is more curved than the vertical meridian. Therefore correction of this astigmatism will require the prescription of convex cylindrical lens at 180° ± 20° and concave cylindrical lens at 90° ± 20° axis.
- *Oblique astigmatism* is a type of regular astigmatism where the two principal meridia are not the horizontal and vertical though these are at right angles to one another (e.g. 45° and 135°). Oblique astigmatism is often found to be symmetrical (e.g. cylindrical lens required at 30° in both eyes) or complementary (e.g. cylindrical lens required at 30° in one eye and at 150° in the other eye).
- *Bioblique astigmatism.* In this type of regular astigmatism the two principal meridia are not at right angle to each other, e.g. one may be at 30° and other at 100°.

4.4.1.3 Optics of regular astigmatism

As already mentioned, in regular astigmatism the parallel rays of light are not focused on a point but form two focal lines. The configuration of rays refracted through the astigmatic surface (toric surface) is called Sturm's conoid and the distance between the two focal lines is known as focal interval of Sturm.

Refractive types of regular astigmatism depending upon the position of the two focal lines in relation to retina, the regular astigmatism is further classified into three types:

- *Simple astigmatism*, where the rays are focused on the retina in one meridian and either in front or behind the retina in the other meridian.
- *Compound astigmatism.* In this type the rays of light in both the meridia are focused either in front or behind the retina and the condition is labelled as compound myopic or compound hypermetropic astigmatism, respectively.
- *Mixed astigmatism* refers to a condition wherein the light rays in one meridian are focused in front and in other meridian behind the retina. Thus in one meridian eye is myopic and in another hypermetropic. Such patients have comparatively less

symptoms as "*circle of least diffusion*" is formed on the retina.

4.4.1.4 Symptoms

Symptoms of regular astigmatism include:

- Defective vision.
- Blurring of objects.
- Depending upon the type and degree of astigmatism, objects may appear proportionately elongated.
- Asthenopic symptoms, which are marked especially in small amount of astigmatism, consist of a dull ache in the eyes, headache, early tiredness of eyes and sometimes nausea and even drowsiness.

4.4.1.5 Signs

- Different power in two meridia is revealed on retinoscopy or autorefractometry.
- Oval or tilted optic disc may be seen on ophthalmoscopy in patients with high degree of astigmatism.
- Head tilt. The astigmatic patients may (very exceptionally) develop a torticollis in an attempt to bring their axes nearer to the horizontal or vertical meridians.
- Half closure of the lid. Like myopes, the astigmatic patients may half shut the eyes to achieve the greater clarity of stenopaeic vision.

4.4.1.6 Investigations

- Retinoscopy reveals different power in two different axis.
- *Keratometry*. Keratometry and computerized *corneal topotograpy* reveal different corneal curvature in two different meridia in corneal astigmatism.
- Astigmatic fan test and Jackson's cross cylinder test. These tests are useful in confirming the power and axis of cylindrical lenses.

4.4.1.7 Treatment

① Optical treatment of regular astigmatism comprises the prescribing appropriate cylindrical lens.

- Spectacles with full correction of cylindrical power and appropriate axis should be used for distance and near vision.
- Contact lenses. *Rigid contact lenses* may correct up to 2~3 D of regular astigmatism, while soft contact lenses can correct only little astigmatism. For higher degrees of astigmatism *toric contact lenses* are needed. In order to maintain the correct axis of toric lenses, ballasting or truncation is required.

② Surgical correction of astigmatism is quite effective.

4.4.2 Irregular Astigmatism

It is characterized by an irregular change of refractive power in different meridia. There are multiple meridia which admit no geometrical analysis.

4.4.2.1 Etiological types
- *Curvatural irregular astigmatism* is found in patients with extensive corneal scars or *keratoconus*.
- *Index irregular astigmatism* due to variable refractive index in different parts of the crystalline lens may occur rarely during maturation of cataract.

4.4.2.2 Symptoms of irregular astigmatism
- Defective vision.
- Distortion of objects.
- Polyopia.

4.4.2.3 Investigations
- Placido's disc test reveals distorted circles.
- Photokerotoscopy and computerized corneal topography give photographic record of irregular corneal curvature.

4.4.2.4 Treatment
- Optical treatment of irregular astigmatism consists of contact lens which replaces the anterior surface of the cornea for refraction.
- Phototherapeutic keratectomy (PTK) performed with excimer laser may be helpful in patients with superficial corneal scar responsible for irregular astigmatism.
- Surgical treatment is indicated in extensive corneal scarring (when vision does not improve with contact lenses) and consists of penetrating keratoplasty.

4.5 ANISOMETROPIA

The optical state with equal refraction in the two eyes is termed isometropia. When the total refraction of the two eyes is unequal, the condition is called anisometropia. Small degree of anisometropia is of no concern. A difference of 1 D in two eyes causes a 2% difference in the size of the two retina images. A difference up to 5% in retinal images of two eyes is well tolerated. In other words, an anisometropia up to 2.5 D is well tolerated and that between 2.5 D and 4 D can be tolerated depending upon the individual sensitivity. However, if it is more than 4 D, it is not tolerated and is a matter of concern.

4.5.1 Etiology
- Congenital and developmental anisometropia occurs due to differential growth of the two eyeballs.
- Acquired anisometropia may occur due to uniocular aphakia after removal of cataractous lens or due to implantation of IOL of wrong power.

4.5.2 Clinical Types
- Simple anisometropia. One eye is normal (emmetropic) and the other either

myopic (simple myopic anisometropia) or hypermetropic (simple hypermetropic anisometropia).
- Compound anisometropia. Both eyes are either hypermetropic (compound hypermetropic anisometropia) or myopic (compound myopic anisometropia), but one eye is having higher refractive error than the other.
- Mixed anisometropia. One eye is myopic and the other is hypermetropic. This is also called antimetropia.
- Simple astigmatic anisometropia. One eye is normal and the other has either simple myopic or hypermetropic astigmatism.
- Compound astigmatic anisometropia. Both eyes are astigmatic but of unequal degree.

4.5.3 Status of Binocular Vision in Anisometropia

Three possibilities are there:
- *Binocular single vision* is present in small degree of anisometropia.
- *Uniocular vision.* When refractive error in one eye is of high degree, that eye is suppressed and develops anisometropic amblyopia. Thus, the patient has only uniocular vision.
- *Alternate vision* occurs when one eye is hypermetropic and the other myopic. The hypermetropic eye is used for distant vision and myopic for near.

4.5.4 Diagnosis

It is made after retinoscopic examination in patients with defective vision.

4.5.5 Treatment

- Spectacles. The corrective spectacles can be tolerated up to a maximum difference of 4 D. After that there occurs diplopia.
- Contact lenses are advised for higher degrees of anisometropia.
- Aniseikonic glasses are also available, but their clinical results are often disappointing.
- Other modalities of treatment include: a. Intraocular lens implantation for uniocular aphakia. b. Refractive corneal surgery for unilateral high myopia, astigmatism and hypermetropia. c. Removal of clear crystalline lens for unilateral very high myopia (Fucala's operation).

4.6 ANISEIKONIA

Aniseikonia is defined as a condition wherein the images projected to the visual cortex from the two retinae are abnormally unequal in size and/or shape. Up to 5% aniseikonia is well tolerated.

4.6.1 Etiological Types
- Optical aniseikonia may occur due to either inherent or acquired anisometropia of high degree.
- Retinal aniseikonia may develop due to displacement of retinal elements towards the nodal point in one eye due to stretching or *oedema* of the retina.
- Cortical aniseikonia implies *asymmetrical* simultaneous perception in spite of equal size of images formed on the two retina.

4.6.2 Clinical Types
Clinically, aniseikonia may be of different types:

1) *Symmetrical* aniseikonia
- *Spherical*. Image may be magnified or minified equally in both meridia.
- *Cylindrical*. Image is magnified or minified symmetrically in one meridian.

2) Asymetrical aniseikonia
- Prismatic. Image difference increases progressively in one direction.
- Pincushion. Image distortion increases progressively in both directions, as seen with high plus correction in aphakia.
- Barrel distortion. Image distortion decreases progressively in both directions, as seen with high minus correction.
- Oblique distortion. The size of image is same, but there occurs an oblique distortion of shape.

4.6.3 Symptoms
- Asthenopia, i.e. eyeache, browache and tiredness of eyes.
- *Diplopia* due to difficult binocular vision when the difference in images of two eyes is more than 5%.
- Difficulty in depth perception.

4.6.4 Treatment
- Optical aniseikonia may be corrected by aniseikonic glasses, contact lenses or intraocular lenses depending upon the situation.
- Retinal aniseikonia treats the cause.
- Cortical aniseikonia is very difficult to treat.

Chapter 5
Optics & Refraction

INTRODUCTION
PHYSICAL OPTICS
GEOMETRIC OPTICS
- ▶ Light Ray
- ▶ Reflection and Refraction of Light
- ▶ Critical Angle and Total Internal Reflection
- ▶ Lens Imaging and Magnification

STATIC RETINOSCOPY
- ▶ Purpose
- ▶ Principle
- ▶ Equipment
- ▶ Setup
- ▶ Procedure
- ▶ Recording

AUTO-REFRACTION
SUBJECTIVE REFRACTION
- ▶ Monocular Subjective Refraction
- ▶ Binocular Balance
- ▶ Recording

5.1 INTRODUCTION

At present, optics can be divided into physical optics, geometric optics and quantum optics according to phenomena. Physical optics describes the wave of light; geometric optics describes the imaging properties of lens and mirrors; quantum optics deals with the interaction of material and light. In this chapter we will focus on physical optics and geometric optics.

Refraction is employed to describe the process of measuring a patient's refractive error and determining the optical correction needed to focus light rays from distant and near objects onto the retina and provide the patient with clear and comfortable vision. During a comprehensive eye examination, your doctor uses refraction to determine how much power is needed to bring your eyes to normal, perfectly focused vision. Your doctor will decide if glasses, contact lenses or laser vision correction will yield you the clearest *eyesight*. The manual determination of the *refractive state* of the eye is an essential and fundamental skill for the student of clinical *ophthalmology* to learn. This outline is designed as a first-order initial orientation to be read as you begin your clinical work. It is far from a thorough manual on the subject, and not a source of theory.

5.2 PHYSICAL OPTICS

Physical optics deals with *coherence* and *diffraction* of light. In physics, the essence of light is electromagnetic radiation, also called *electromagnetic wave*. It is a specific *wavelength*, according to the wavelength of short to long, can be divided into γ-rays, X-rays, *ultraviolet*, visible light, *infrared* and radio waves. Visible light is only a tiny fraction of electromagnetic waves, lies between ultraviolet and infrared portions, from 380 nm at the violet end of the *spectrum* to 760 nm at the red end. The visual receptors in our retinas (cone-rod) respond only to this part of the electromagnetic wave and ignore other wavelengths. A single wavelength of visible light will produce *monochromatic* light. Different colours are excited by light of different wavelengths. It will produce seven colors: violet, indigo, blue, green, yellow, orange and red (*Table 5-1*). Seven monochromatic lights mixed in a certain proportion will produce white light.

Table 5-1 The relationship between visible light wavelength and color vision

Color Vision	Visible Light Wavelength(nm)	Color Vision	Visible Light Wavelength(nm)
red	780~620	blue	490~450
orange	620~590	indigo	450~430
yellow	590~560	violet	430~380
green	560~490		

In a *vacuum*, the speed of all wavelengths of light is the same, that is, $c=3.0\times10^8$ m/s (The exact value is 299 792 458 m/s). In other mediums, such as air, water, glass, etc., light travels more slowly. The ratio of the speed of light in a vacuum(c) to the speed in the medium(v) is called the *refractive index* (n) of the medium. The higher the index, the slower the speed.

$$n = c / v$$

The speed and wavelength of light can be changed in different optical media, but frequency is constant. Color depends on frequency, so that the color of the light is not altered as it passes through optical media except by selective non-transmittance or fluorescence.

5.3 GEOMETRIC OPTICS

Geometrical optics, or ray optics, describes light *propagation* in terms of "rays". The "ray" in geometric optics is an abstraction or "instrument", which can be used to approximately model how light will propagate. Light rays bend at the interface between two dissimilar media, and may curve in a medium where the refractive index changes. Geometrical optics provides rules for propagating these rays through an optical system. The path taken by the rays indicates how the actual wave will propagate. This is a significant simplification of optics that fails to account for optical effects such as *diffraction* and *polarization*. It is a good approximation, however, when the wavelength is very small compared with the size of structures which the light interacts. Geometric optics can be used to describe the geometrical aspects of imaging. It is essential to understand the optics of eye, refraction errors and their correction.

5.3.1 Light Ray

Light ray is a line or curve that is *perpendicular* to the light's *wavefronts* (and is therefore *collinear* with the *wave vector*), and indicates the direction in which light travels. A slightly more rigorous definition of a light ray follows from Fermat's principle, which states that the path taken between two points by a ray of light is the path that can be traversed in the least time. A collection of countless rays of light that are related to each other is called a beam of light. There are four types of beams: *convergent* beams, *divergent* beams, *parallel* beams, and *astigmatic* beams (*Figure 5-1*).

5.3.2 Reflection and Refraction of Light

The laws of *reflection* and *refraction* were formulated in 1621 by the Dutch astronomer and mathematician Willebrod Snell at the University of Leyden. These laws, together with Fermat's principle, form the basis of applied geometric optics. They can all be stated as follows (*Figure 5-2*).

5.3.2.1 Reflection of light

When light hits a surface, or the interface between two media, some of it is reflected. The light rays falling on a reflecting surface are called incident rays and those reflected by it are reflected rays. A line drawn at 90 angle to the surface is called the surface normal (or normal). The law of reflection is independent of the wavelength, the material of the medium and the incident angle of light.

Laws of reflection are:

- The *incident ray,* the *reflected ray* and the normal are in the same plane.
- The angle of incidence(θ_1) is equal to the angle of reflection(θ_2).

Glossy surfaces such as *plane mirrors* reflect light in a simple, predictable way, called *specular reflection* (*Figure 5-3*). This allows for production of reflected images that can be associated with an actual (*real image*) or extrapolated (*virtual image*) location in space. For *flat mirrors*, the law of reflection implies that images of objects are upright and the same distance behind the mirror as the objects are in front of the mirror. The image size is the same as the object size. (The *magnification* of a flat mirror is unity.) The law also implies that mirror images are parity inverted, which we perceive as a left-right inversion.

If a beam of light hits a *rough surface*, each ray of light still follows the law of reflection, but each reflected ray goes in a different direction. This phenomenon is called *diffusion* (*Figure 5-4*).

5.3.2.2 Refraction of light

Refraction of light is the phenomenon of change in the path of light, when it goes from one medium to another at any angle other than 90° or 0°. The light rays falling on the *interface* between two media are called incident rays and those refracted by it are refracted rays. A line drawn at 90 angle to the surface is called the normal. The basic cause of refraction is light travels at different speeds from one medium to the other. Refraction of light is the most commonly observed phenomenon. For example, if we put a chopstick into the water, it will appear that the chopstick is bent upwards. In fact, the chopstick is still straight, but the light is bent.

Laws of refraction (*Figure 5-5*) are :
- The incident ray, the refracted ray are on opposite sides of the normal and all the three are in the same plane.
- The angle of incidence θ_1 is related to the angle of refraction θ_2. To be more specific, the product of the index of refraction of the medium of the incident ray (n_1) and the sine of the angle of incidence of the incident ray ($\sin\theta_1$) is equal to the product of the same terms of the refracted ray ($n_2, \sin\theta_2$) : $n_1 \sin\theta_1 = n_2 \sin\theta_2$. This law is also called Snell's law.

5.3.3 Critical Angle and Total Internal Reflection

From Snell's law, when light goes from an optically less-dense medium (air, n_1) to an optically denser medium (glass/water, n_2), the angle of refraction is less than the angle of incident ($\theta_2 < \theta_1$). Conversely, when light goes from an optically denser medium (n_2) to an optically less-dense medium (n_1), the angle of refraction is greater than the angle of incident ($\theta_2 > \theta_1$). In this situation, as the angle of incidence is increased, *the critical angle* is reached when the light is totally reflected. (The angle of refraction is 90° and there is actually no refraction, only the angle of reflection.) If the light enters at an angle greater than critical angle, the ray is totally reflected back into the denser medium, and it will not be refracted,

which is called *total internal reflection*. From the above, two conditions must be met for total internal reflection to occur:
- The incident light must be directed from an optically denser medium (n_2) to an optically less-dense medium (n_1).
- The incident angle must be greater than the critical angle.

Total internal reflection obeys the laws of regular reflection, being utilized in many optical equipment, such as fiber optics, applanation *tonometer*, and indirect *ophthalmoscopy*.

5.3.4 Lens Imaging and Magnification

A device which produces converging or diverging light rays due to refraction is known as a lens. Thin lenses produce *focal points* on either side that can be modeled using the lensmaker's equation. In general, two types of lenses exist: *convex lenses*, which cause parallel light rays to converge, and *concave lenses*, which cause parallel light rays to diverge. The detailed prediction of how images are produced by these lenses can be made using ray-tracing similar to curved mirrors. Similarly to curved mirrors, thin lenses follow a simple equation that determines the location of the images given a particular *focal length* (f) and object distance (S_1):

$$\frac{1}{S_1} + \frac{1}{S_2} = \frac{1}{f}$$

where S_2 is the distance associated with the image and is considered by convention to be negative if on the same side of the lens as the object and positive if on the opposite side of the lens. The focal length f is considered negative for concave lenses.

Incoming parallel rays are focused by a convex lens into an inverted real image one focal length from the lens, on the far side of the lens. Rays from an object at finite distance are focused further from the lens than the focal distance. The closer the object is to the lens, the further the image is from the lens. With convex lenses, incoming parallel rays diverge after going through the lens, in such a way that they seem to have originated at an upright virtual image one focal length from the lens, on the same side of the lens that the parallel rays are approaching on. Rays from an object at finite distance are associated with a virtual image that is closer to the lens than the focal length, and on the same side of the lens as the object. The closer the object is to the lens, the closer the virtual image is to the lens.

Likewise, the magnification of a lens is given by

$$M = \frac{S_1}{S_2} = \frac{f}{f - S_1}$$

where the negative sign is given, by convention, to indicate an upright object for positive values and an inverted object for negative values. Similar to mirrors, upright images produced by single lenses are virtual while inverted images are real.

Lenses suffer from *aberrations* that distort images and focal points. These are due to both geometrical imperfections and the changing index of refraction for different wavelengths of light (*chromatic aberration*).

5.4 STATIC RETINOSCOPY

The procedure of determining and correcting refractive errors is termed as refraction. The refraction is a dynamic, multi-procedural clinical diagnostic process. The refraction comprises two complementary methods, objective and subjective. An objective refraction is a refraction obtained without receiving any feedback from the patient. However, a subjective refraction requires responses from the patient.

One of the most common instruments used for objective refraction is the retinoscope. Using a retinoscope, your doctor will project a streak of light into your pupil. A series of lenses are flashed in front of your eye. By looking through the retinoscope, your doctor can study the light reflex of the pupil. Based on the movement and orientation of this retinal reflection, the refractive state of your eye is measured. There are two types of retinoscopes, a "spot" and a "streak" retinoscope, and the "streak" is the one you will learn to use here.

5.4.1 Purpose

Examiners should determine the distance refractive status of the patient's eyes objectively. The results of this technique can be used as a starting point for the *subjective refraction* or as the patient's final prescription. (If the patient is unable to respond to subjective testing.)

5.4.2 Principle

Retinoscopy is based on the fact that when light is reflected from a mirror into the eye, the direction in which the light will travel across the pupil will depend on the refractive state of the eye.

The retinoscope uses the retinoscopy mirror's illumination system to illuminate the interior of the eyeball, and the light is reflected from the retina. The reflected light changes after passing through the refraction component of the eyeball, which can be used to determine the refractive state of the eye (*Figure 5-6*).

5.4.3 Equipment
- Streak *retinoscopy.*
- *Phoropter*, lens rack, or loose trial lenses. The technique described here refers to lenses in the phoropter because that is the usual clinical method of retinoscopy. The same principles can be applied to retinoscopy using loose lenses or a retinoscopy rack instead of the phoropter.
- Fixation target: 20/400 E projected through a red/green filter.

5.4.4 Setup

- The patient removes his corrective lenses.
- Adjust the height of the examination chair so that the patient's eyes are at the same level as the doctor.
- *Disinfect* patient contact surfaces of the phoropter by wiping it with alcohol.
- Place the phoropter in front of the patient with the *pupillary distance (PD)* set to match the patient's distance PD. Level the phoropter so the patient's eyes are centered in the apertures.
- Instruct the patient to keep both eyes open during retinoscopy. Ask the patient to inform the doctor if doctor's head blocks his view of the fixation target. It may be necessary to rotate the phoropter slightly or to move the target off the screen and onto the wall.
- During retinoscopy, the doctor should keep both eyes open and examine the patient's right eye with his right eye and the patient's left eye with his left eye.
- The doctor holds the retinoscope 50 cm or 67 cm from the patient's eyes. The retinoscope is held in the doctor's right hand to examine the patient's right eye and left hand to examine the patient's left eye.
- Retinoscopy is most easily done in dim *illumination*. Generally, start by turning off all the lights.

5.4.5 Procedure

① Turn on the retinoscope light and make sure the sleeve of the streak retinoscope is in the "down" position.

② Instruct the patient to look at the fixation target and examine the patient's right eye.

③ Determine if the refractive error is spherical or astigmatic by changing the position of the sleeve of the streak retinoscope and the distance between the doctor and the patient until the reflex is enhanced. Then rotate the streak of the retinoscope through 360° looking for the break phenomenon, the thickness phenomenon, the skew phenomenon, or changes in the brightness of the reflex within the pupil.

- If the error is spherical, the reflex within the pupil will be continuous with the intercept of the streak on the patient's face. If the error is astigmatic, the reflex within the pupil may not be continuous with the intercept on the patient's face.
- As the streak is rotated through 360°, the thickness of the reflex within the pupil will be constant in a spherical error and vary in an astigmatic error. Moreover, as the streak is rotated, the brightness of the pupillary reflex will remain constant in a spherical error and may vary in an astigmatic error. The principal meridians correspond to the orientations of the streak that provide the thickest and thinnest reflexes and/or the brightest and dimmest reflexes and the orientation of the streak in which the reflex within the pupil is exactly continuous with the intercept of the

streak on the patient's face.
- In an astigmatic error, as the streak is swept across the patient's pupil, the reflex within the pupil will move parallel to the movement of the streak on the patient's face when the streak is aligned with one of the two principal meridians. The reflex will move in a different direction than the streak when the streak is not aligned with one of the principal meridians. There will be no skew phenomenon in a spherical error.

④ When the motion of the reflex is in the same direction as the sweeping motion of the light across the pupil, it is known as *with motion*. Conversely, when the motion of the reflex is in the opposite direction as the sweeping motion of the light across the pupil, it is known as *against motion*. If the error is spherical, observe the reflex for with or against motion and add plus or minus lenses until there is no motion of the reflex. The type of lens needed for *neutralization* depends on the patient's refractive error, the position of the sleeve of the retinoscope, and the type of motion seen (*Figure 5-7*).

Note: With motion is easier to observe and to neutralize than against motion. However, if with motion is present, the patient may *accommodate*, particularly if *minus lenses* were added.

⑤ To neutralize an astigmatic error, first identify the two principal meridians. Then neutralize each *meridian* separately. When using a phoropter with minus cylinders, one meridian is neutralized with spherical power only and the other meridian is neutralized with a combination of spherical power and minus cylinder. The least myopic or most hyperopic meridian is neutralized with spherical power. The most myopic or least hyperopic meridian is neutralized with cylinder in addition to the spherical power.

Since it may be difficult for a novice retinoscopist to determine which meridian is the least myopic, either meridian can be neutralized first. Then, another meridian can be checked and adjusted if necessary. If the retinoscopist neutralizes the most myopic meridian first, one meridian will show neutrality while the other shows with motion. To correct this, the retinoscopist can add more plus spherical power to neutralize the second meridian. This will leave the first meridian showing against motion. The newly created against motion can be neutralized by adding minus-cylinder power with the cylinder axis aligned with the orientation of the streak.

It is often observed, particularly when the pupils are large, that the motion of the reflex in the *periphery* of the pupil differs from that observed near the center of the pupil. This is called "scissors motion". For purposes of refraction, the goal is to achieve neutrality at the center of the pupil, ignoring peripheral reflex movements.

⑥ When both principal meridians are neutralized, recheck the meridian neutralized with spherical power and adjust the spherical power if necessary. The lens (or combination of lenses) that produces neutrality is called the "gross retinoscopy finding" or simply the "gross". The gross retinoscopy finding makes the patient's fundus conjugate with the doctor's entrance pupil, not optical infinity. Leaving the gross static finding in front of the patient's right eye and neutralize the patient's left eye by following previous steps. When the patient's left eye is neutralized, recheck the left eye and adjust the spherical or cylinder power if necessary.

⑦ To convert the gross retinoscopy finding to a net finding, algebraically add a spherical minus lens equal to your working distance in diopter to the spherical lens that produced neutrality. For example, add −2.00 D for a working distance of 50 cm and −1.50 D for a working distance of 67 cm. This is the "net static retinoscopy finding" or the "net static". The patient's retina focuses with infinity if the retinoscopy is accurate.

⑧ Measure the patient's *visual acuity* in each eye through the net static retinoscopy finding.

5.4.6 Recording

- Record the net static for each eye separately.
- Record the patient's visual acuity for each eye through the net *static retinoscopy* finding.

5.5 AUTO-REFRACTION

Auto-refraction is also called automatic objective refractors, which estimates the refractive error without requiring either doctor or patient judgment. It has been available since 1969. These instruments are easy to operate, quicker than other techniques of objective refraction such as retinoscopy and are better appreciated by patients. For these reasons autorefractors are enjoying an increased popularity in ophthalmologic and optometric practice to objectively assess the refractive error of patients, and in some situations to completely dispense with retinoscopy.

An auto-refractor is a computerized instrument that shines light into your eye. The light travels through the front part of your eye to the back part of your eye, then back again. The information bounces back to the instrument, giving an objective measurement of your refractive error. Auto-refractors are quick and easy to use, and require no feedback from you.

5.6 SUBJECTIVE REFRACTION

Subjective refraction is meant for finding out the most suitable lenses to be prescribed. The goal of the subjective refraction is to achieve clear and comfortable binocular vision. The subjective refraction starts after retinoscopy or autorefraction, which provides the clinician with an objective assessment of refractive error. It is possible to start with the patient's previous prescription; however, this is the least desirable way to begin, as there is no objective information about the patient's current refractive error. Thus, the best starting point is from the objective determination of refractive error by retinoscopy.

Subjective refraction requires responses from the patient. The doctor may use a phoropter to measure patient's subjective refractive error to determine his/her eyeglass prescription. Typically, the patient will sit behind the phoropter and look at an eye chart. The doctor will change lenses and other settings while asking the patient for feedback on which settings give him/her the best vision.

Sometimes eye doctors prefer to obtain a *cycloplegic refraction*, especially when trying to obtain an accurate refraction in young children who may skew refraction measurements by adjusting their eyes. Cycloplegic eye drops are applied to the eye to temporarily paralyze the ciliary muscle of the eye.

The basic steps in performing the subjective properly are always as follows.

5.6.1 Monocular Subjective Refraction
5.6.1.1 Initial MPMVA (maximum plus to maximum visual acuity)

1) Purpose

To determine the maximum plus (minimum minus) spherical power which provides the patient with his maximum *visual acuity (VA)*. The *initial MPMVA* begins with the net static retinoscopy or the auto-refraction.

2) Procedure

① Open the right eye and occlude the left eye.

② Fog the eye to a visual acuity of 20/40 to 20/60. This usually requires adding about +1.00 D to +1.50 D spherical power (or removing −1.00 D to −1.50 D spherical power) to the net static retinoscopy or the auto-refraction. Check the patient's VA through the fogging lenses to ensure he/she is fogged to the correct level.

③ Predict the final spherical power by comparing the patient's VA under fog to Egger's chart. Remember that the patient should obtain approximately one additional line of VA for each −0.25 D spherical power added (or +0.25 D spherical power removed) during the MPMVA.

④ Reduce the plus (or add minus) 0.25 D spherical power at a time, checking VA and encouraging the patient to read the next smaller line each time.

⑤ Keep in mind that each 0.25 D should allow the patient to read smaller letters. If reducing +0.25 D (or increasing −0.25 D) has not improved VA, it indicates that the patient has achieved maximum visual acuity. At a certain point adding more minus will not make the chart any clearer, it will only seem to make the letters smaller (minified). So if they can see 20/20, don't add more minus.

⑥ Reach an appropriate stopping point. To decide when to stop the initial MPMVA, choose one of the following endpoints.
- The bichrome endpoint. The bichrome red-green test was taken as the endpoint. (More details will be provided later.)
- The 20/20 endpoint. If the patient has subjectively clear vision (20/20 or better), and

the lenses in the phoropter at previous steps match the refraction that was predicted from the starting information, the initial MPMVA may be stopped.

Consider the following points:

- Does the amount of minus added correlate with the amount of improvement in VA over the starting point with the patient fogged? The correct refraction will yield a close match between the actual and predicted changes in lens power.
- If the phoropter contains a tentative cylinder of −0.75 D or greater from static retinoscopy or some other test, proceed with the *Jackson cross cylinder test*. Remember that a visual acuity of 20/20, or sharp, clear vision may not be possible at this point in the refraction because the cylindrical part of the refraction has not yet been refined.
- If the static retinoscopy and other starting data do not indicate any astigmatism and the patient does not achieve 20/20 VA or better with spherical lenses, consider the possibility that the eye suffers from pathology (such as opacities in medium) or *amblyopia*.
- If the patient has clear VA of 20/20 or better with spherical lenses and if you are refracting the right eye, proceed to the monocular refraction of the left eye. Then, proceed to the *binocular balance*.

5.6.1.2 Bichrome red-green test

1) Purpose

To determine the correcting spherical lens power.

The *bichrome red-green test* should be used as the endpoint procedure for the initial MPMVA.

2) Procedure

① Put the projectors red-green filter over the chart of letters.

② Direct the patient's attention to the 20/25 line or to the letters one line above his/her best VA so far. For some patients it may be necessary to isolate this line of letters.

③ Tell the patient to look from the green side to the red side and back to the green side. Ask the patient "Which side has the sharper and clearer letters?" (not better, darker, or brighter) or "Are both sides equally clear?". Since this test works on the principle of chromatic aberration, it will not work for color anomalous patients. For such individuals, it may be necessary to tell them to look at the left or right side of the chart rather than at the green or red side.

- If the letters on the red side are clearer, introduce an additional 0.25 D of minus-spherical power (or take away 0.25 D of plus spherical power).
- If the letters on the green side are clearer, take away 0.25 D of minus spherical power (or add another 0.25 D of plus spherical power).

④ Repeat the previous steps until you find the minimum minus power (or maximum plus) at which the patient reports slightly clearer green side letters. As an alternative, use a red-green balance, the point at which both sides appear equally clear, rather than one into the green, as the endpoint.

⑤ Remove the red-green filter and recheck the VA.

Note: Some patients are unresponsive to this test and seem to choose one side or the other regardless of the lenses powers in place. Be alert to this possibility and abandon the bichrome red-green test in favor of some other endpoint to the MPMVA.

5.6.1.3 The Jackson cross cylinder (JCC) test

The JCC is a single lens that is a combination of a plus and minus cylinder. The one in the phoropter is a +0.25 D and a −0.25 D cylinder. The red dots are the axis of the minus cylinder, and the white dots are the axis of the plus cylinder. While testing axis, you need to "straddle" the correcting cylinder with the axis of the JCC. In other words, the red dots and the white dots should be 45° from the correcting cylinder.

Ordinarily, we should refine cylinder axis first then power using the Jackson cross cylinder(JCC). However, if the tentative cylinder power is only −0.50 D or −0.25 D, it is preferred to perform power check prior to axis. If the patient accepts the cylinder power at this time, the axis check followed by refinement of the cylinder power with the refined cylinder axis in place. If the patient rejects the cylinder power at this time, do the second MPMVA.

1) Purpose

To refine the axis and power of the cylindrical component of the refraction after the initial monocular MPMVA has determined the tentative spherical refraction.

2) Procedure of the JCC axis check

① Flip the JCC and ask the patient which side is clearer. Tell him/her that both views may be blurry, but he/she will tell you which view is sharper or less blurry. Further instructs him/her to try to ignore differences in the shapes of the letters when comparing the views.

② If the views are not equally blurry or equally clear, move the axis of the phoropter cylinder by 10° toward the minus-cylinder axis (indicated by the red marks) that gives the clearer view. If view number 1 provides the patient with clearer vision, the axis in the phoropter should be moved in a clockwise direction. If view number 2 provides the patient with clearer vision, the axis in the phoropter should be moved in a counterclockwise direction.

③ Shift the orientation of the JCC lens so that the handle or thumb wheel remains aligned with the axis of the phoropter cylinder. In many phoropters, the JCC will rotate automatically along with the phoropter cylinder, so this step is unnecessary.

④ Repeat previous steps as long as you have to keep adjusting the cylinder axis in the same direction. When the axis has to be moved in the opposite direction, repeat previous steps, but move the axis in 5° steps. Hone in on the correct axis by successively decreasing the step size.

Note: The greater the cylinder power, the greater the need for precision in the axis. For cylinder powers greater than 5.0 D, the axis should be specified to the single degree. For cylinder powers less than 2.0 D, the axis should be specified to the nearest 5°. For cylinder powers between 2.0 D and 5.0 D, exercise professional judgment.

End the JCC axis check when either of the following two conditions are met:
- Both views look the same to the patient.
- The patient's responses move the axis back and forth within a narrow range. In this event, select an axis in the middle of the range or at or close to the axis in the patient's habitual lens prescription.

3) Procedure of the JCC power check

① Turn the JCC 45° so that the dots line up with the correcting cylinder axis. Now as you flip the JCC, you will either be adding −0.50 cylinder or taking away −0.50 D cylinder.

② Flip the JCC. When the red dots are lined up with the correcting cylinder axis, you are increasing corrective cylinder power. Conversely, when the white dots are lined up, you are taking away corrective cylinder power.

③ Ask the patient "Which is better, one or two?". Their preference will direct you towards increasing or decreasing the corrective cylinder.

④ If their response directs you to add cylinder, add one half of a diopter. If their response directs you to decrease cylinder, decrease by one half of a diopter. When the responses to the JCC flip are equivocal (equal blur on both sides of the flip), you have theoretically arrived at the correct cylinder amount.

Note: Always keep the spherical equivalent constant when changing cylinder powers. The purpose is to keep the astigmatic interval straddling the retina, which is necessary for valid astigmatic testing (theoretical explanation to come). This is done by changing the sphere power by half the amount of the cylinder change in the opposite direction. For example, if you increase the corrective cylinder by −0.50 D cylinder, change the sphere by +0.25 D sphere. And if you take away −0.50 D cylinder, change the sphere by −0.25 D sphere.

End the JCC power check when either of the following two conditions are met:
- Both views look equally clear or equally blurry to the patient.
- The patient's responses call for changes within a narrow range of powers. In this event, select the power that is closer to that found in his habitual prescription. If a habitual prescription is not available, select the lesser minus-cylinder power.

Note: For some patients, making the choice of which view is clearer is very difficult. Borish describes a variation on the JCC technique in which the whole VA chart, from the 20/50 to 20/15 letters, rather than an isolated line of letters, is displayed. The patient is asked to report which view allows him/her to read farther down the chart. By having the patient try to read the chart, the examiner can exercise his/her professional judgment as to the view that provides the sharper retinal image.

Upon reaching the conclusion of the JCC test for both axis and power, perform the second monocular MPMVA.

Chapter 5 Optics & Refraction

5.6.1.4 Second monocular MPMVA

If the JCC test has not changed the cylinder axis and power or there is no astigmatism in the initial data, only the initial MPMVA is required. If changed, you need to do the second monocular MPMVA, go back and retest the best spherical power. The procedure and endpoint of the second monocular MPMVA are the same as the initial MPMVA.

Repeat previous steps with the left eye occluded and the left eye open.

5.6.1.5 Clock chart (astigmatic fan)

The clock chart (also called astigmatic fan) is performed if 20/20 VA cannot be achieved with spherical lenses and the starting points of the refraction indicate a need for cylinder. It is also indicated if there is reason to believe that the tentative cylindrical correction from the static retinoscopy is inaccurate. Clock chart is done one eye at a time.

The astigmatic fan consists of a dial of lines radiating at 10° or 15° interval to one another (*Figure 5-8*). The emmetropic patient will see all the lines equally clear. In the presence of astigmatism, some lines will be seen more sharply defined. The concave cylinder is then added with its axis at right angles to the clearest line until all the lines are equally sharp.

1) Purpose

To determine the cylinder axis and power of the refractive error by a subjective technique.

2) Procedure

① Occlude the eye not being tested.

② Remove any cylinder that may have been in the phoropter and fog the eye being tested to a VA of 20/40 with spherical lenses.

③ Show the patient the clock chart.

④ Ask the patient to identify the darkest, sharpest set of lines in the clock chart according to their position on the face of a clock.

- If all the lines appear equally blurry, the test did not detect any uncorrected astigmatism and the test is terminated.
- If one set of lines appears clearer or darker than the others, set the axis of the minus cylinder in the phoropter to 30 times the smaller o'clock from the patient's report. This is known as the "rule of 30".
- If two sets of lines seem about equally dark or sharp, select an axis value midway between.

⑤ Gradually add −0.25 D cylinder power. Each time, ask the patient if one set of lines is clearer or darker than the others, until the patient reports that all of the lines look equally clear or blurry.

5.6.2 Binocular Balance

Since this binocular balance procedure calls upon the patient to match the VA under fog in the two eyes, perform it only if the two eyes achieve the same VA during their monocular refraction. If the best corrected VA of the two eyes differ after the distance monocular subjective refraction, the binocular balance procedure should be skipped.

To equalize the stimulus to accommodation for the two eyes. The primary purpose of binocular balance is to match the accommodative stimulus for the two eyes. It serves a secondary purpose of relaxing the accommodation. With both eyes open, the accommodative responses of the two eyes should be maximally relaxed and equal. For many patients, binocular balance serves the additional function of matching the visual acuity in the two eyes through the new prescription.

5.6.2.1 Prism dissociated test

① Make sure that neither eye is occluded and that both eyes can see the projector screen.

② Fog each eye by +0.75 D spherical power relative to the endpoint of its respective monocular refraction. Measure the patient's binocular VA and continue adding +0.25 D spherical power in front of both eyes until the binocular VA is 20/25 or worse, if necessary.

③ Isolate a line of letters one line above the VA found at the end of previous steps.

④ Place 3△ to 4△ base up over the right eye and 3△ to 4△ base down over the left eye using the phoropter's *rotary (Risley) prisms*.

⑤ Inform the patient that he/she should see two lines of letters, both of which should be blurry. Make certain that this is the case.

⑥ Ask the patient to look back and forth between the two lines of letters and have him/her tell you which line, the upper or the lower, is clearer or less blurry.

⑦ Add +0.25 D (take away −0.25 D) spherical power to the eye which sees the clearer line. For example, if the patient reports that the lower line is clearer, add +0.25 D spherical power to the right eye.

⑧ Repeat previous steps until the patient reports equal blurriness of the two lines or the patient is simply switching back and forth between the two. If it is not possible to achieve a close match between the blurriness of the two eyes, perform the sighting dominance check. Then leave the *sighting-dominant eye* with the subjectively clearer vision.

⑨ When equality of the vision of the two eyes is reached, or the sighting-dominant eye is left with the slightly clearer vision, remove the Risley prisms to allow *fusion*.

5.6.2.2 Prism-dissociated bichrome test

① Make sure neither eye is occluded and both eyes can see the visual acuity chart on the screen.

② Isolate a line of letters one line above the VA of the poorer eye at the end of the monocular subjective refraction. Fogging lenses are not added.

③ Place the red-green filter over the isolated line of letters.

④ Using the phoropters Risley prisms, place 3△ to 4△ BU over the right eye and 3△ to 4△ BD over the left eye.

⑤ Inform the patient that he/she should see two lines of letters on a red or green background. Make certain that this is the case.

⑥ Direct the patient's attention to the lower line of letters, which are seen by the right eye. Tell him/her to look from the green side to the red side and back to the green side. Ask him/her to state which side has the sharper, clearer letters (not better, darker, or brighter) or to state if the two sides are equally clear.

⑦ If the letters on the red side are clearer or the two sides are equally clear, introduce an additional 0.25 D of minus spherical power (or take away another 0.25 D of plus) in front of the right eye. If the green side are clearer, take away 0.25 D of minus (or add another 0.25 D of plus) in front of the right eye.

⑧ Direct the patient's attention to the upper line of letters and repeat previous steps on the left eye.

⑨ Repeat the previous steps until you find the minimum minus power (or maximum plus) at which the patient reports a slightly clearer green side letters, for both the upper and the lower line letters. As an alternative endpoint, use a red-green balance, the point at which both sides appear equally clear, rather than one into the green.

⑩ Remove the red-green filter and recheck the VA in each eye separately and in both together.

Note: Some patients always seem to choose either the red or the green side regardless of the lens powers in place. Be alert to the possibility that your patient is unresponsive to the bichrome test and abandon it in favor of the smaller/darker endpoint for each eye separately.

5.6.2.3 Binocular MPMVA

To determine the maximum plus-spherical power which provides the patient with maximum visual acuity through both eyes simultaneously.

Binocular MPMVA is performed on the basis of binocular balance. After binocular balance, the prism is removed and binocular MPMVA is performed. That is to say, both eyes are defogged to reach the end of optometry. The procedure and endpoint of the binocular MPMVA are the same as the monocular MPMVA, except that the detection is done when both eyes are fixed simultaneously.

5.6.3 Recording

Record the sphere power, cylinder power, and cylinder axis in the phoropter for each eye. Measure and record the VA for the right eye, the left eye, and for both eyes together.

Note: The patient's final eyeglass prescription may differ from the results of the distance subjective refraction with the phoropter. Some examples will illustrate this point. If the prescription is greater than ± 4.0 D, it is necessary to adjust it for the vertex distances of the phoropter versus the patient's spectacles. Be conservative about changing the cylindrical components (particularly the axis) of a prescription that is comfortable for the patient. For high amounts of cylinder, it may be necessary to prescribe a different axis and power in glasses that will be used for reading as opposed to distance viewing.

Chapter 6
Accommodation and Vergence

INTRODUCTION
- Accommodation
- Vergence
- Relationship Between Accommodation and Vergence

ACCOMMODATIVE DYSFUNCTION
- Accommodative Insufficiency
- Ill-Sustained Accommodation
- Accommodative Infacility
- Paralysis of Accommodation
- Spasm of Accommodation

VERGENCE DYSFUNCTION
- Convergence Insufficiency
- Divergence Excess
- Basic Exophoria
- Convergence Excess
- Divergence Insufficiency
- Basic Esophoria
- Fusional Vergence Dysfunction
- Vertical Heterophorias

MANAGEMENT
- Basis for Treatment
- Available Treatment Options
- Patient Education
- Prognosis and Follow-up

Chapter 6 Accommodation and Vergence

6.1 INTRODUCTION

6.1.1 Accommodation

Accommodation is the process by which the *vertebrate* eye changes optical power to maintain a clear image (focus) on an object as its distance changes. Accommodation acts like a reflex, but can also be consciously controlled. *Mammals,* birds and *reptiles* vary the optical power by changing the form of the elastic lens using the ciliary body (in humans up to 15 diopters). Fish and *amphibians* vary the power by changing the distance between a rigid lens and the retina with muscles.

The young human eye can change focus from distance to 7 cm from the eye in 350 milliseconds. This dramatic change in focal power of the eye of approximately 12 diopters (a diopter is 1 divided by the focal length in meters) occurs as a consequence of a reduction in *zonular* tension induced by ciliary muscle contraction. The amplitude of accommodation declines with age. By the fifth decade of life the *accommodative amplitude* has declined so the *near point* of the eye is more remote than the reading distance. When this occurs, the patient is presbyopic. Once *presbyopia* occurs, those who are *emmetropic* (do not require optical correction for distance vision) will need an optical aid for near vision; those who are myopic (*nearsighted* and require an optical correction for distance vision) will find that they see better at near without their distance correction; and those who are hyperopic (*farsighted*) will find that they may need a correction for both distance and near vision. The age-related decline in accommodation occurs almost universally, and by 60 years of age, most of the population will have noticed a decrease in their ability to focus on close objects.

The most widely held theory of accommodation is that proposed by Hermann von Helmholtz in 1855. When focusing at near the circular muscle fibers of the ciliary muscle contract, decreasing the equatorial *circumlenticular* space which reduces zonular tension and allows the lens to round up and increase in optical power. When viewing a distant object, the circular ciliary muscle fibers relax which increases the *equatorial* circumlenticular space, causing an increase in zonular tension. The increase in zonular tension causes the surface of the lens to flatten and the optical power of the lens to decrease.

6.1.2 Vergence

A *vergence* is the simultaneous movement of both eyes in opposite directions to obtain or maintain single binocular vision. When a creature with binocular vision looks at an object, the eyes must rotate around a vertical axis so that the projection of the image is in the center of the retina in both eyes. To look at an object closer by, the eyes rotate towards each other (convergence), while for an object farther away they rotate away from each other (divergence). Exaggerated convergence is called cross eyed viewing (focusing on the nose for example). When looking into the distance, the eyes diverge until parallel, effectively fixating the same point at *infinity* (or very far away).

Vergence movements are closely connected to accommodation of the eye. Under normal conditions, changing the focus of the eyes to look at an object at a different distance will automatically cause vergence and accommodation.

6.1.3 Relationship Between Accommodation and Vergence

It is normally accompanied by a convergence of the eyes to keep them directly at the same point, sometimes termed accommodation convergence reflex.

When someone accommodates to a near object, they also converge their eyes and constrict their pupils. The combination of these three movements (accommodation, convergence and miosis) is under the control of the Edinger-Westphal nucleus and is referred to as the *near triad*. Although it is clear that convergence allows to focus the object's image on the retina, the functional role of the pupillary contraction remains less clear. Arguably, it may increase the depth of field by reducing the aperture of the eye, and thus reduce the amount of accommodation needed to bring the image in focus on the retina.

There is a measurable ratio between how much convergence takes place because of accommodation (AC/A ratio, CA/C ratio). Abnormalities with this can lead to many *orthoptic* problems.

6.2 ACCOMMODATIVE DYSFUNCTION

This book uses the Duke-Elder classification of *accommodative dysfunction*.

6.2.1 Accommodative Insufficiency

Accommodative insufficiency occurs when the amplitude of accommodation (AA) is lower than expected for the patient's age and is not due to *sclerosis* of the crystalline lens. Patients with accommodative insufficiency usually demonstrate poor accommodative sustaining ability.

6.2.2 Ill-Sustained Accommodation

Ill-sustained accommodation is a condition in which the AA is normal, but *fatigue* occurs with repeated accommodative stimulation.

6.2.3 Accommodative Infacility

Accommodative infacility or accommodative inertia occurs when the accommodative system is slow in making a change, or when there is a considerable lag between the *stimulus* to accommodation and the accommodative response. The patient often reports blurred distance vision immediately following sustained near work. Some have considered this infacility to be a *precursor* to myopia.

6.2.4 Paralysis of Accommodation

Paralysis of accommodation is a rare condition in which the accommodative system fails to respond to any stimulus. It can be caused by the use of cycloplegic drugs, or by trauma, ocular or systemic disease, toxicity, or poisoning. The condition, which can be unilateral or bilateral, may be associated with a fixed, *dilated* pupil.

6.2.5 Spasm of Accommodation

The result of overstimulation of the *parasympathetic nervous* system, *spasm of accommodation* may be associated with fatigue. It is sometimes part of a triad (overaccommodation, overconvergence, and miotic pupils) known as spasm of the near reflex (SNR). This condition may also result from other causes, such as the use of either systemic or topical cholinergic drugs, trauma, brain tumor, or myasthenia gravis.

6.3 VERGENCE DYSFUNCTION

The classification of *vergence dysfunction* is based on a system originally developed by Duane for application to *strabismus*. The system has been modified for the classification of heterophoria and *intermittent strabismus*.

6.3.1 Convergence Insufficiency

"Classic" *convergence insufficiency (CI)* consists of a receded *near point of convergence (NPC)*, exophoria at near, reduced positive fusional convergence (PFC), and deficiencies in negative relative accommodation (NRA). However, not all patients with CI have all of these clinical findings. CI can be described as a deficiency of PFC relative to the demand and/or a deficiency of total convergence, as measured by the NPC; it has been called "common CI".

6.3.2 Divergence Excess

Divergence excess (DE) can be described clinically as exophoria or exotropia at far greater than the near deviation by at least 10 prism diopters (PD). Divergence excess can be further divided into true or simulated DE on the basis of responses to occlusion. In simulated DE, occlusion dramatically affects slow vergence, increasing the angle of deviation slightly at distance and significantly at near. Occlusion does not affect true DE.

6.3.3 Basic Exophoria

The patient with *basic exophoria* has a deviation of similar magnitude at both distance and near.

6.3.4 Convergence Excess

The patient with *convergence excess (CE)* has a near deviation at least 3 PD more esophoric than the distance deviation. The etiology of the higher esodeviation at near most commonly is indicated by a high accommodative convergence/accommodation (AC/A) ratio.

6.3.5 Divergence Insufficiency

In a patient with *divergence insufficiency (DI)*, tonic *esophoria* is high when measured at distance but less at near. Symptomatic patients usually have low fusional divergence amplitudes at distance and low AC/A ratios.

6.3.6 Basic Esophoria

The patient with *basic esophoria* has high tonic esophoria at distance, a similar degree of esophoria at near, and a normal AC/A ratio.

6.3.7 Fusional Vergence Dysfunction

Patients with *fusional vergence dysfunction* (vergence insufficiency) often have normal phorias and AC/A ratios but reduced fusional vergence amplitudes. Their zone of clear, *single binocular vision (CSBV)* is small.

6.3.8 Vertical Heterophorias

Vertical heterophorias may be either *comitant* and idiopathic or noncomitant, due to muscle *paresis* or other mechanical cause. One of the most common causes of newly acquired vertical diplopia or *asthenopia* with vertical deviation is longstanding, decompensated, fourth nerve palsy, which results in superior oblique paresis. These patients demonstrate a *hyperphoria* in primary gaze that is initially greatest during depression and *adduction* of the affected eye. Over time, secondary overaction and contracture of the inferior oblique muscle may overshadow the initial fourth nerve palsy. Thus, the deviation may be largest during elevation and adduction of the affected eye.

6.4 MANAGEMENT

Management of the patient with an accommodative or vergence dysfunction is based on interpretation and analysis of the examination results.

6.4.1 Basis for Treatment

The general goals for the treatment and management of accommodative and/or vergence dysfunction are:
- To assist the patient to function efficiently in school performance, at work, and/or in athletic activities.

- To relieve ocular, physical, and psychological symptoms associated with these disorders.

6.4.1.1 Vision therapy

1) Accommodative therapy

The purpose of accommodative therapy is to increase the amplitude, speed, accuracy, and ease of accommodative response. At the end of therapy, the patient should be able to make rapid accommodative responses without evidence of fatigue.

Several studies have reported that accommodation can be modified with therapy. Repeated accommodative testing itself improves accommodative responses. Studies have also shown that voluntary accommodation can be taught and that accommodation skills developed by biofeedback can transfer from one task to another.

Research has demonstrated the effectiveness of accommodative therapy in eliminating decreased accommodative amplitude and facility. In one study, 87% of the patients with accommodative anomalies had eliminated their asthenopia and normalized their accommodative findings after approximately 26 therapy sessions. Therapy to improve AA can result in a concurrent improvement of PFC, NFV, and *stereopsis*. Vision therapy is the method of choice in eliminating asthenopic symptoms associated with accommodative anomalies. For those patients who cannot participate in vision therapy, plus lenses may successfully decrease symptoms.

In a double-blind prospective study to determine the effects of monocular AA therapy on asthenopia, the patients in the experimental group had dramatically improved AA, reduced accommodative time constants, and significantly reduced symptoms. None of these changes was evident in the control group. When the control group underwent therapy identical to that received by the experimental group, a similar reduction in symptoms and normalization of accommodative function was achieved.

These studies suggest that vision therapy is effective in altering accommodation, with a resultant change in amplitude and facility and a decrease in symptoms. Therapy can also result in positive changes in the magnitude, velocity, and gain of the accommodative response. Accommodative therapy not only eliminates symptoms but is associated with objective changes in the velocity of the accommodative response and a concurrent decrease in recorded time constants. Therapy improves the time characteristics, including both latency and velocity of the accommodative response.

2) Vergence therapy

Fusional vergence therapy improves slow vergence (vergence adaptation) ; thus, it reduces the apparent vergence error. This reduction in the residual vergence error apparently causes a change in the AC/A ratio. Other important functions of slow vergence include maintenance of fusion following blinking, reduction of the fusional demand with the *onset* of presbyopia, and maintenance of *binocularity* when age and diseases such as *hyperthyroidism* have altered *orbital* contents. If the vergence and accommodative systems are functioning properly when a steady-state level of accommodation or vergence is reached, the slow accommodation and vergence systems maintain accommodation and vergence without effort. The fast and slow vergence and accommodative systems also use proximal, tonic, and voluntary vergence and accommodation to reduce their loads. Defects in any one of these systems alone may not result in asthenopia or strabismus, owing to overlap with components in other systems.

Numerous studies have evaluated the effectiveness of vergence therapy in eliminating subjective and objective findings associated with binocular anomalies. These studies demonstrate that vergence therapy improves vergence ability, and that the effects persist over time. All of the studies demonstrating the efficacy of vision therapy used in-office therapy regimens.

Vision therapy for vergence dysfunction has a high success rate. Pooled data for patients with CI indicate that 72% of patients have been successfully managed, while 19% improved significantly and only 9% failed. Vision therapy has a lasting effect when a complete cure is achieved. Moreover, age is not a deterrent in the successful management of binocular anomalies.

A controlled, *prospective*, double-blind, A-B reversal study compared vergence treatment and *placebo* treatment in a group of patients diagnosed with CI. *Random dot stereograms* were presented in an operant conditioning paradigm to improve vergence amplitudes. The experimental group had dramatic improvement in vergence amplitudes and concurrent decrease in symptoms. When the control group crossed over to become the experimental group, the findings were similar.

The convergence insufficiency treatment trial (CITT) comprised two pilot studies and one large clinical trial. In the first clinical trial, 47 children 9~17 years of age with symptomatic CI were randomly assigned to office-based vision therapy, office-based placebo vision therapy, or home-based pencil push-up therapy. Symptoms were significantly reduced in the vision therapy group but not in the pencil push-up or placebo vision therapy groups. Only patients in the vision therapy group demonstrated both statistically and clinically significant changes in near point of convergence and positive fusional vergence at near. Neither pencil push-ups nor placebo vision therapy was effective in improving either symptoms or signs associated with convergence insufficiency.

Adults 19~34 years of age were evaluated using an identical *protocol* to that of the children's study. At the end of therapy, the CI symptom survey showed a significant reduction in symptoms for patients in each of the three treatment groups. However, patients in the vision therapy group had the greatest reduction in symptoms. Patients treated with pencil push-ups and placebo vision therapy did not achieve normal symptom scores.

Two hundred and twenty-one 9 to 17-year-olds with symptomatic CI participated in the full CITT *clinical trial*. The four management strategies included active vision therapy, computerized home therapy, placebo vision therapy, and push-ups. At the end of 12 weeks of therapy, there was a reduction in symptoms for patients in each of the four treatment groups. Patients in the vision therapy group had the greatest reduction in symptoms. Those in the pencil push-up, computerized home therapy, and placebo vision therapy groups did not achieve normal symptom scores. Over time, trends showed a reduction in symptoms for all groups. These studies indicate that vision therapy results in a clinical and statistical reduction in symptoms that is not due to placebo effects.

All CITT groups showed an improvement in the NPC. Over time, the office-based vision therapy group showed the greatest changes, followed by the home computerized vision therapy, pencil push-ups, and placebo therapy groups. Follow-up at 6 months and 1 year after 12 weeks of therapy showed no regression from the post treatment results for any of the four management strategies. Thus, post-therapy effects persist for at least 1 year.

A retrospective study evaluated 43 presbyopic patients with presumed symptomatic vergence anomalies who completed a home computerized vision therapy program. The authors concluded that when in-office vision therapy is not practical, patients who demonstrate symptoms associated with an accommodative/vergence anomaly may use a home computerized therapy system.

The pooled success rates of different treatment regimens for *intermittent* exotropia have been reported as: 59% for vision therapy, 46% for surgery, and 28% for passive therapy (minus lenses, occlusion, and/or prisms). These data suggest that vision therapy is more effective than surgery in patients with intermittent exotropia.

A study evaluating the use of vision therapy in 31 intermittent exotropia patients reported that 64.5% were classified as cured; 9.7%, improved; and 9%, fair. A follow-up study found that after 5 years, 52% of these patients remained cured, while 32% were in the improved group. Similar findings have been reported by other studies. One study reported that the highest success rate occurred when in-office therapy was supplemented with home vision therapy.

An additional study to demonstrate the effectiveness of vision therapy for CE, treated 68 patients diagnosed with CE. Total elimination of symptoms occurred in 80% of the patients. Among the improvements achieved with vision therapy were an increase in mean divergence amplitude from 8 PD to 16 PD, an increase in recovery value from 2 PD to 10 PD, and increased *accommodative facility* from 1.5 to 8 cycles per minute. Prior to therapy, some subjects had been prescribed spectacles to eliminate the esophoria; others had not. Comparison of the results for the patients receiving vision therapy alone with the results for patients initially receiving reading spectacles and then undergoing vision therapy showed no difference in the post-vision therapy results, suggesting that vision therapy alone is highly effective in eliminating abnormal vergence findings associated with CE.

6.4.1.2 Lens and prism therapy

1) Horizontal prisms

Clinicians often prescribe prism to eliminate symptoms of asthenopia and to reduce the fusional vergence demand in patients with vergence dysfunction. Two common methods of determining the amount of prism to prescribe are a. to satisfy Sheard's criteria and b. to eliminate the FD. One study evaluated the effect of prescribing prism, using the associated *heterophoria* to eliminate the FD in three groups of patients: symptomatic exophoric patients, symptomatic esophoric patients, and a control group. Each patient received two pairs of spectacles to be worn for 2 weeks, one pair with a prismatic correction that eliminated the associated phoria and the second pair with no prism. While 73% of the symptomatic exophoric patients and 90% of the symptomatic esophoric patients preferred the prismatic glasses, 86% of the asymptomatic patients rejected the prismatic glasses.

In a prospective double-masked, multicenter, randomized clinical trial, 72 children aged 9 through 17 years with symptomatic CI were randomly assigned to base-in prism glasses or glasses without prism. They were instructed to wear the glasses for all near tasks. The CISS was given at the baseline examination and after 6 weeks of wearing glasses. The BI-prism reading glasses were found to be no more effective than placebo reading glasses in alleviating symptoms or improving the near point of convergence or positive fusional vergence at near in the children with symptomatic CI. These results demonstrate the potentially powerful placebo effect of prescribing any eyeglasses for children 9 through 17 years old.

A prospective study of symptomatic CI subjects aged 45~68 years was performed; whereby each subject was assigned two pairs of progressive addition glasses, one with BI prism and one without prism. The subjects wore each pair of glasses for 3 weeks and then completed the CISS. The mean CISS score of 30 at baseline decreased to 13 with the BI-prism glasses and to 24 with glasses without prism. Progressive addition glasses with BI prism were found to be effective in reducing symptoms of presbyopes with symptomatic CI, at least for the short term.

Prism may be the only viable treatment for CI in patients who are unable to participate in a vision therapy program because of time, or cognitive or financial constraints; however, it should be used with caution. Although patients with symptomatic vergence anomalies may be treated with prisms, adaptation to prismatic correction limits its effectiveness. Slow vergence (prism or vergence adaptation) varies from patient to patient. It also varies with the amount of time spent wearing the prism, the power or strength of the prism, and the direction of prism placement (e.g. base-out, base-up). When prism adaptation occurs, prism therapy is contraindicated for two reasons: a. the prism will not permanently neutralize the deviation, and b. strong vergence adaptation will not be able to handle the stress placed on the vergence system by the heterophoria. Only when there is a significant deviation with minimal vergence adaptation can prism compensation be effective.

Adaptation to base-out and base-in prisms differs. As expected, most people adapt faster and more completely to BO prism than to BI prism. Prolonged wearing of prisms not only alters the heterophoria position, but also results in a readjustment of horizontal fusional amplitudes. Once adaptation has occurred, measurements of the fusional vergence amplitudes, with the prism in place, are almost identical to the measurements prior to wearing the prism. Most of this change occurs within the first 15 minutes of wearing the prism.

Vergence adaptation also occurs with noncomitant deviations. The phenomenon of adaptation, a continuous process that can occur over the entire oculomotor field, explains why patients who wear incorrectly centered ophthalmic lenses or *anisometropic* prescriptions may not complain. Many patients adapt to a newly introduced prism, and its abrupt removal may result in diplopia and/or asthenopia. Symptomatic patients who do not adapt to prisms usually report a reduction in asthenopia once they wear a prism prescription.

2) Vertical prisms

Vertical deviations may be divided into three different categories: small-angle comitant deviations; large-angle, newly acquired paretic deviations; and large-angle, *decompensated*, older deviations. Studies have shown that patients with these deviations differ in their adaptation responses to vertical prism. Although the adaptation process varies from individual to individual, in general, the larger the prism, the less complete the adaptation process. The longer the prism is worn, the more complete the adaptation process and the longer the recovery after removal of the prism. Patients who do not show significant adaptation may benefit from prism correction.

Clinically, adaptation can be determined by having the patient wear a vertical prism for as little as 1~2 hours. Adaptation can be predicted to occur whenever a heterophoria increases dramatically after repeated, prolonged cover testing. The effectiveness of prism is limited by torsional deviations, noncomitancies, and anisometropia. Surgery or vision therapy may be needed to supplement prismatic correction.

3) Plus lenses

The purpose of plus lenses is to decrease the demand on the accommodation system and/or to reduce the amount of the esodeviation by manipulating the crosslink AC/A ratio. Adaptation does seem to play a significant role in the prescription of plus lenses. The effectiveness is limited in patients who demonstrate accommodative dysfunction with asthenopia in the absence of a large heterophoria, and in those whose accommodative and fusional amplitudes are constricted but equal (i.e., PRA/NRA).

4) Minus lenses

Minus lenses may be used to change the motor demand of the vergence system by reducing the amount of exodeviation.

5) Surgery

The purpose of extraocular surgery is to decrease the size of the deviation; therefore, it is rarely indicated for nonstrabismic binocular vision disorders. One study advocates surgical intervention for CI when vision therapy fails; however, the study did not have a large enough sample to support the author's conclusion concerning the use of surgery as a primary mode of treatment for CI.

Surgery may be considered for cases of noncomitant vertical deviations that have a significant torsional component. Newly acquired large-angle vertical deviations that cannot be resolved within 6 months may require surgery. As a general rule, vision therapy alone is ineffective in treating newly acquired large-angle vertical deviations. If the patient is satisfied with prismatic correction or vision therapy, surgical intervention is not necessary.

6.4.2 Available Treatment Options

Treatment and management of accommodative and vergence anomalies are designed to eliminate signs and symptoms such as headaches, asthenopia, poor academic performance, poor job performance, loss of concentration, and ocular and systemic fatigue. Because it also eliminates other symptoms such as diplopia, reduced stereopsis, and motion sickness, treatment and management generally improves the patient's quality of life.

Treatment options can be divided into the following broad categories: optical correction, including added lens power and prism; vision therapy; pharmaceutical agents; and *extraocular muscle* surgery. Therapeutic results can vary due to differences in the application of the specific treatment regimen.

6.4.2.1 Optical correction

1) Ophthalmic lenses

Appropriate spectacle lens correction of any existing refractive error is the first consideration in treating persons with vergence or accommodative anomalies. Plus lenses are often effective in eliminating symptoms in the patient who has an accommodative insufficiency or imbalanced positive and negative relative accommodative values. In addition, plus lenses may positively affect abnormal esophorias according to the AC/A ratio.

Plus additions at near may be used for the patient diagnosed with an accommodative anomaly or with an abnormally high AC/A ratio. Lens power may be determined by many different methods: balancing the PRA and NRA values; cross-cylinder; near point retinoscopy; or calculation of the AC/A ratio to determine the minimum lens power that can significantly reduce the near deviation.

2) Prisms

Prisms are often effective in eliminating vergence disorder symptoms that involve a significant motor deviation (tonic vergence anomaly).

Horizontal prisms—Sheard's criterion can be used to calculate the amount of prism required to alleviate symptoms using the following formula:

$$\text{Prism power} = \frac{2 \times \text{heterophoria} - \text{opposing vergence}}{3}$$

Other methods of prescribing prism include using Percival's criterion, in which the clinician prescribes prism to place Donder's line in the middle third of the graph in graphical analysis, and FD methods, in which the clinician prescribes the amount of prism that eliminates the FD (i.e. the linear associated phoria).

Vertical prisms—There are three types of vertical deviations: a. longstanding, asymptomatic deviations that have very strong vergence adaptation; b. longstanding deviations that decompensate and have moderate vergence adaptation; and c. recent, small deviations with minimal vergence adaptation. Each of these vertical deviations requires a different prismatic correction. Patients with old deviations that decompensate usually present with minimal symptoms in relation to the size of the deviation. The prismatic correction needed to eliminate or reduce symptoms is usually minimal compared with the magnitude of the deviation. On the other hand, the patient who has a newly acquired hyperdeviation with minimal vergence adaptation may require full prism correction, which is defined as the amount of prism needed to correct either the heterophoria or the recovery value. Patients who have strong vergence adaptation and are asymptomatic usually should not be treated with prism.

6.4.2.2 Vision therapy

Three general phases of vision therapy will be discussed in this section: accommodation, vergence, and accommodative/vergence interaction. This book will use the term "vision therapy" rather than similar terminology such as "vision training" or "orthoptics".

The first phase of therapy is to normalize accommodative and vergence amplitudes. Most clinicians use large targets to slowly change convergence and divergence demand. The patient is encouraged to exert maximum effort to increase his or her vergence amplitudes. Accommodative facility exercises are performed concurrently.

The second phase of accommodative and vergence therapy is designed to increase the speed of response to accommodative and vergence stimuli. During this phase, it is beneficial to use targets that gradually become smaller and to use different stimuli to obtain generalization. After the amplitudes reach normal levels, the patient is encouraged to repeat the task enough times to make the response become automatic and effortless. Once monocular accommodative facility has improved, binocular accommodative facility procedures can be performed. Suppression controls may be needed with the binocular accommodative techniques. In general, the power of the binocular accommodative flippers is increased until the patient can successfully clear +/−2.50 D, according to a specified criterion.

The third phase of vision therapy uses jump or step vergence stimuli. Instead of responding to incrementally increasing stimuli, the patient is required to make large-jump accommodative and vergence movements. Finally, accommodation and vergence are integrated through techniques that stimulate accommodation while holding vergence stable and vice versa. This final phase of vision therapy is designed to automate both accommodative and vergence reflexes.

Vision therapy increases the magnitude and the velocity of the fast fusion system. In addition, there is a concurrent increase in both the magnitude and velocity of the slow vergence system (vergence adaptation). In a study to evaluate the effect of vision therapy on vergence adaptation, subjects who underwent 8 weeks of vision therapy that consisted of push-ups and fusional amplitude therapy had improved vergence adaptation and fusional amplitudes. Subsequent studies have demonstrated that vision therapy alters the fixation disparity curve (FDC), specifically, flattening the FDC and concurrently reducing the symptoms.

The success of vision therapy lies in the improvement of both the accommodative and vergence adaptation systems, because these systems are the most important for a person's long-term comfort. Although the patient may have a normal fast vergence system, he or she may have an abnormal slow vergence system, with the resulting symptoms. Thus, therapy is first aimed at improving reflex-fast fusional vergence, then at expanding slow vergence responses. In the process, accommodative flexibility is also restored. The last stage of therapy enhances the flexibility between accommodation and vergence. The goal of vision therapy is to re-establish automated, effortless accommodative and vergence responses under any stimulus condition. Improvement of amplitudes alone is not sufficient.

There is a paucity of data demonstrating the efficacy of using home based vision therapy alone. If in-office therapy is not available, home computerized vision therapy with push-ups should be offered as an alternative.

6.4.2.3 Surgery

Extraocular muscle surgery is rarely advocated to treat nonstrabismic vergence defects. As a general rule, it should be considered only when optical correction or vision therapy methods have failed and a significant heterophoria continues to produce symptoms. There is no surgery available for accommodative dysfunction.

6.4.3 Patient Education

Patients should be advised that many accommodative and vergence anomalies are neuromuscular problems and not refractive problems. Thus, the most effective treatment relies on not only spectacles, but also active vision therapy to eliminate neuromuscular dysfunction. Patients should also be told that treatment improves accommodative and vergence reflexes. Proper management usually results in improvement, due to changes in the slow vergence system.

6.4.4 Prognosis and Follow-up

When the patient is cooperative, the *prognosis* for the elimination of accommodative and vergence dysfunction is excellent. The most effective treatment appears to be in-office vision therapy, supplemented by home therapy. Prisms and lenses may be less effective in eliminating some vergence dysfunctions. The difficulty with lenses is that they do not affect either the fast vergence or slow vergence systems. Furthermore, the effectiveness of prisms and lenses may be reduced by adaptation. These options will only be effective if there is significant heterophoria or an inability to sustain accommodation.

Patients with accommodative and convergence problems who have been treated successfully should be seen twice a year for the first year, then annually thereafter. Patients for whom spectacles are prescribed to eliminate symptoms of asthenopia should be followed as necessary. Many practitioners schedule a *follow-up visit* after the patient has worn his/her prescribed spectacles for 1 month and again 3~6 months later.

Chapter 7
Spectacles

INTRODUCTION
SPECTACLE FRAME
  ▶ The Classification of Spectacle Frames
  ▶ Spectacle Frame Selection
LENSES
  ▶ The Materials
  ▶ The Surface Treatment
TINTED LENSES AND PHOTOCHROMATIC LENSES
CORRECTIVE LENSES
  ▶ Single Vision Lenses
  ▶ Bifocals, Trifocals, and Progressive Multifocal Lenses
  ▶ Peripheral Defocus Lenses
  ▶ Pinhole Glasses
SAFETY GLASSES
SUNGLASSES
3D GLASSES
READING GLASSES

7.1 INTRODUCTION

Spectacles (also called *eyeglasses* or *glasses*) are *frames* bearing lenses worn in front of the eyes, a kind of optical device, normally for vision correction or eye protection (such as protection from UV rays, ocular trauma). It is a common, cheap and easy method of prescribing corrective lenses in patients with refractive errors and presbyopia. Not all glasses are designed solely for vision correction but are worn for protection, viewing visual information (such as stereoscopy or simply just for *aesthetic* or fashion values). *Safety glasses* are a kind of eye protection against flying debris or against visible and near visible light or *radiation*. Sunglasses allow better vision in bright daylight, and may protect against damage from high levels of ultraviolet light.

The lenses fitted in a frame constitute spectacles. Modern glasses are typically supported by *nose pads* on the bridge of the nose and by temple arms placed over the ears. Historical types include the *pince-nez*, *monocle*, *lorgnette*, and scissors-glasses.

7.2 SPECTACLE FRAME

Spectacles are the daily necessities for aesthetic needs. The significance and function of spectacle frame have far exceeded the original intention of being an eyeglass carrier, and also give consideration to the functions of comfort, safety and beauty.

7.2.1 The Classification of Spectacle Frames

According to the national classification standard of spectacle frames released in 2003, spectacle frames can be divided into metal frames, plastic frames, natural material frames and mixed frames according to materials. On the basis of style, it can be divided into full frame, *semi-rimless frame,* rimless frame, combination frame and folding frame.

The earliest spectacle frames are made of *natural materials* such as stones, *crystals* and animal bones. Hawksbill and buffalo horn are rare natural materials, rich in color and beautiful texture. Some also have health care functions. These materials are as sophisticated as diamond-cutting techniques and commonly used to make high-end luxury frames.

Since the 18th century, metal materials have been the mainstay of spectacle frames, often made of single metal or alloy materials, such as nickel alloy, copper alloy, titanium alloy, and precious metal. Currently, the most common metal frame uses pure titanium, memory metal titanium alloy, high nickel alloy, etc. They are strong, beautiful, light, corrosion-wear resistance, easy to process, but the price is relatively high.

Plastic frames are favored by consumers because they are light, fashionable and easy to match clothes, mainly with cellulose nitrate (CN), cellulose acetate (CA), cellulose propionate (CP), cellulose acetate butylate (CB), polycarbonate(PC), epoxy resin, and polyamide as raw material. The full name of TR90 is "Grilamid TR90", also known as memory nylon, is derived from the improvement of polyamide as raw material, and has been widely used in recent years. It is light, strong, impact resistance, wear resistance, high temperature resistance, etc., especially suitable for the production of sports and children's spectacle frames.

7.2.2 Spectacle Frame Selection

In addition to functionality and aesthetics, the most important thing in spectacle frame selection is comfortable, neither tight nor loose, light in weight and should not put pressure on the nose or temples of the patient, and should be of optimum size. In children, large glasses are recommended to prevent viewing over the spectacles. Ideally, the lenses should be worn 15.3 mm from the cornea (the anterior focal plane of eye), as at this distance the images formed on the retina are of the same size as in emmetropia.

7.3 LENSES

A lens is a transparent refracting medium, bounded by two surfaces which form a part of a sphere (spherical lens) or a cylinder (toric or astigmatic lens). Toric or astigmatic lenses are prescribed to correct astigmatism, bounded by at least one cylinder surface. Spherical lenses are bounded by two spherical surfaces and are mainly of two types: convex (plus lens) and concave (minus lens). Concave lens is used for correction of myopia and convex lens is used for correction of hypermetropia, presbyopia or aphakia. Aphakia literally means absence of *crystalline lens* from the eye. However, from the optical point of view, it may be considered a condition in which the lens is absent from the pupillary area. Aphakia produces a high degree of hypermetropia.

The power of a lens is generally measured in diopters. Convex lenses have negative diopter strengths; concave lenses have negative diopter strengths. Prescription lenses, made to conform to the prescription of an *ophthalmologist* or *optometrist*, are used to make prescription glasses, which are then verified correct using a professional lens meter.

Modern lenses are made up of different materials and coatings with optical and chemical properties. The materials and surface treatment are closely related to the vision, comfort, durability and safety of the lens.

7.3.1 The Materials

Crown glass of refractive index 1.5223 is very commonly used for spectacles. It is ground to the appropriate curvature and then *polished* to await the final cutting that will enable it to fit the desired spectacle frame.

Plastic lenses, including CR-39 and *polycarbonate* are unbreakable and light weight. These materials reduce the danger of breakage and weigh less than glass lenses. Some plastics also have more advantageous optical properties than glass, such as better transmission of visible light and greater absorption of ultraviolet light. Some plastics have a greater index of refraction than most types of glass; this is useful in the making of corrective lenses shaped to correct various vision abnormalities such as myopia, allowing thinner lenses for a given prescription. Newer plastic lenses can also correct for the *higher order aberrations* that naturally occur on the surface of the eye. These lenses create sharper vision for people who have problems with sight.

CR-39 lenses are the most common plastic lenses due to their low weight, high scratch resistance, and low transparency for ultraviolet and infrared radiation. Polycarbonate lenses are the lightest and most shatter-resistant, making them the best for impact protection, though polycarbonate offers poor optics due to high dispersion, having a low *abbe number* of 31.

7.3.2 The Surface Treatment

Scratch-resistant coatings can be applied to most plastic lenses, giving them similar scratch resistance to glass. *Hydrophobic coatings* designed to ease cleaning are also available, as are *anti-reflective coatings* (AR coatings) intended to reduce *glare*, improve night vision and make the wearer's eyes more visible.

7.4 TINTED LENSES AND PHOTOCHROMATIC LENSES

Tinted glasses reduce the amount of light they transmit and provide comfort, safety and cosmetic effects. They are particularly prescribed in patients with *albinism,* high myopia and glare prone patients. Good tinted glasses should be dark enough to absorb 60% ~80% of the incident light in the visible part of the spectrum and almost all of the ultraviolet and infrared rays.

Photochromatic lenses, which are photosensitive, darken when struck by UV light. These lenses do not function efficiently indoors and in automobiles.

7.5 CORRECTIVE LENSES

7.5.1 Single Vision Lenses

Single vision lenses refer to lenses having the same corrective power over the entire surface. These are used to correct refractive errors of the eye by modifying the effective focal length of the lenses in order to alleviate the effects of conditions such as nearsightedness (myopia), farsightedness (hyperopia) or astigmatism. Another common condition in older patients is presbyopia which is caused by the eye's crystalline lens losing elasticity, progressively reducing the ability of the lens to accommodate (i.e. to focus on objects close to the eye).

Over the years, these lenses have increased in sophistication and are now made in many brands and variations, with extremely complex design formulations, to produce bifocals, trifocals, *progressive multifocal lenses*, and peripheral defocus lenses.

7.5.2 Bifocals, Trifocals, and Progressive Multifocal Lenses

As people age, their ability to focus is lessened and many decide to use *multiple-focus lenses*, which can be *bifocal*, *trifocal* or even progressive multifocal (*Figure 7-1),* to cover all the situations in which they use their sight. Traditional multifocal lenses have two or three distinct horizontal viewing areas, bifocal lenses have different powers to upper (for distant vision) and lower (for near vision) segments; trifocal lenses have three portions, upper (for distant vision), middle (for intermediate range vision) and lower (for near vision). Some modern multifocal lenses, such as progressive lenses (known as "no-line bifocals"), give a smooth transition between these different focal points, unnoticeable by most wearers, while other glasses have lenses specifically intended for use with computer monitors at a fixed distance.

7.5.3 Peripheral Defocus Lenses

Investigations have shown that myopic eyes often exhibit relative hyperopia in the periphery, and it has been suggested that the hyperopic defocus at the retinal periphery may act as a signal for increased eye growth.

Peripheral defocus lenses (*Figure 7-2*) designs were intended to reduce peripheral hyperopic defocus and inhibit the axial growth of the eye. It may be possible to slow the progression of myopia by altering the curvature of the image shell at the same time as the central refractive error is corrected, thereby either partly or fully correcting any hyperopic defocus at the periphery or even inducing peripheral myopic defocus.

7.5.4 Pinhole Glasses

Pinhole glasses are a type of corrective glasses which do not use a conventional lens and are claimed to help correct the eye's refractive error without introducing the image distortion of traditional lens-based glasses.

Pinhole glasses, especially multiple-pinhole glasses,can be used for correction of presbyopia, as well as near and distance vision correction irrespective of an individual's refraction status. A small aperture in the pinhole glasses narrows the incident ray, blocks aberrant rays from reaching the retina, and ultimately increases the clarity of retinal images. This pinhole effect enhances the depth of focus and amplitude of accommodation. Therefore, pinhole glasses can improve visual acuity in individuals.

7.6 SAFETY GLASSES

Safety glasses (*Figure 7-3*) are usually made with shatter-resistant plastic lenses to protect the eye from flying debris. Although safety lenses may be constructed from a variety of materials of various impact resistance, certain standards suggest that they maintain a minimum 1 mm thickness at the thinnest point, regardless of material. Safety glasses can vary in the level of protection they provide. For example, those used in medicine may be expected to protect against blood *splatter* while safety glasses in a factory might have stronger lenses and a stronger frame with additional *shields* at the temples. The lenses of safety glasses can also be shaped for correction.

The American National Standards Institute has established standard ANSI Z87.1 for safety glasses in the United States, and similar standards have been established elsewhere.

Some safety glasses are designed to fit over corrective glasses or sunglasses. They may provide less eye protection than *goggles* or other forms of eye protection, but their lightweight increases the likelihood that they will actually be used. Modern safety glasses tend to be given a more stylish design in order to encourage their use. Corrective glasses with plastic lenses can be used in place of safety glasses in many environments; this is one advantage that they have over contact lenses.

There are also safety glasses for *welding*. These are often called "flash goggles", because they provide protection from welding flash.

Worker safety eyewear is available in various lens colors and/or with coatings to protect or enable eyesight in different lighting conditions, particularly when outdoors.

Nylon frames are usually used for protection eyewear for sports because of their lightweight and flexible properties. They are able to bend slightly and return to their original shape instead of breaking when pressure is applied to them. Nylon frames can become very brittle with age and they can be difficult to adjust.

7.7 SUNGLASSES

Sunglasses may be made with either prescription or non-prescription lenses that are darkened to provide protection against bright visible light and, possibly, ultraviolet (UV) light. Light *polarization* is an added feature that can be applied to sunglasses lenses. Polarization filters remove horizontally polarized rays of light, which eliminates glare from horizontal surfaces.

Yellow lenses increase color contrast and improve depth perception. Brown lenses are common among golfers, but cause color distortion. Also, green/yellow tinted lenses are common when night driving and aid in the removing of glare off on-coming headlights. Blue, purple, and green lenses offer no real benefits to vision enhancement, and are mainly cosmetic. Some sunglasses with interchangeable lenses have optional clear lenses to protect the eyes during low light or night time activities and a colored lens with UV protection for times where sun protection is needed.

Sunglasses are often worn just for aesthetic purposes, or simply to hide the eyes. Many blind people wear *opaque* glasses to hide their eyes for aesthetic reasons.

7.8 3D GLASSES

The *illusion* of three dimensions on a two dimensional surface can be created by providing each eye with different visual information. Classic 3D glasses (*Figure 7-4*) create the illusion of three dimensions when viewing specially prepared images. The classic 3D glasses have one red lens and one blue or cyan lens. Another kind of 3D glasses uses *polarized filters*, with one lens polarized vertically and the other horizontally, with the two images required for *stereo vision* polarized the same way. Polarized 3D glasses allow for color 3D, while the red-blue lenses produce a dull black-and-white picture with red and blue fringes. Both types have been distributed to audiences at 3D movies.

7.9 READING GLASSES

Magnifying lenses (*Figure 7-5*) or generic spectacles that are used to treat mild presbyopia can be bought off the shelf. It is usually composed of a convex lens, a frame and a handle. Although such glasses are generally considered safe, an individual prescription, as determined by an ophthalmologist or optometrist and made by a qualified optician, usually results in better visual correction.

Chapter 8
Contact Lenses

HISTORY OF CONTACT LENSES
PHYSIOLOGY OF THE HUMAN EYE
- ▶ The Origin of Eyes
- ▶ Structure of Eyes

PROPERTIES OF CONTACT LENS MATERIALS
- ▶ Chemical Properties
- ▶ Mechanical Properties
- ▶ Optical Properties

CONTACT LENS MANUFACTURE
- ▶ Molding
- ▶ Lathe Cutting

NOMENCLATURE FOR CONTACT LENS
- ▶ Diameters of the Lens
- ▶ Curves of the Lens
- ▶ Edge of the Lens
- ▶ Power of the Lens
- ▶ Thickness of the Lens
- ▶ Tint

TYPES OF CONTACT LENS
- ▶ Hard Lenses
- ▶ Rigid Gas Permeable Lenses (RGP)
- ▶ Soft Lenses
- ▶ Corrective Contact Lenses
- ▶ Cosmetic Contact Lenses
- ▶ Therapeutic Contact Lenses
- ▶ Some Other Types

THE APPLICATION OF CONTACT LENSES
- ▶ Advantages of Contact Lenses over Spectacles
- ▶ Contraindications for Contact Lens Use
- ▶ Indications of Contact Lens Use

8.1 HISTORY OF CONTACT LENSES

- Leonardo da Vinci introduced the concept of contact lenses in 1508, followed by René Descartes in 1636.
- The first pair of contact lenses was manufactured by Thomas Young in 1801. John Herschel conceived the possibility to obtain molds of the cornea by impression on a transparent material.
- In 1888, Adolf Fick successfully constructed and fitted *scleral lenses* for the first time. They were made of heavy blown glass, with *diameters* ranging from 18 to 21 mm. Fick's lenses were fitted on rabbits and on human volunteers using a *dextrose solution*, and they allowed a maximum wearing time of 2 h.
- The development of Plexiglas in the 1930s allowed to manufacture plastic contact lenses. Contact lenses made of fully plastic materials were produced by István Györffy in 1939.
- *Polymethyl methacrylate (PMMA)* corneal lenses gained popularity in the 1960s.
- Upon realizing that the low oxygen *permeability* of PMMA was the cause of several *adverse effects*, from the 1970s *Rigid Gas Permeable (RGP)* materials were introduced. In 1965, Bausch & Lomb started to manufacture contact lenses with *hydrogels* in the US, previously invented by Wichterle and Lím in 1959. The first hydrogel contact lenses appeared in the 1960s, and in 1971 the Soflens material received the first FDA approval.
- In 1972, *disposable* soft contact lenses were produced.
- The first *silicone* hydrogel contact lenses were successfully manufactured in 1998. Silicone hydrogels combined high oxygen permeability and wearing comfort. Diverse commercial materials with similar properties followed shortly after.
- Nowadays, silicone hydrogels and RGP materials lead the market of soft and rigid lenses, respectively. A timeline on the history of contact lenses is illustrated in Figure 8-1.

8.2 PHYSIOLOGY OF THE HUMAN EYE

8.2.1 The Origin of Eyes

The first reported eye-like structure dates back to 521 million years ago, during the cambrian explosion, in which earth has seen the first optical devices in animals in the form of eyes with lenses, followed by the first reflector around 13 years later.

In the same period, a variety of life forms started differentiating from the worm-like animals that inhabited earth until then to most of the phyla known today, and visual systems quickly became a dominant arm in the survival game. Optical structures found in animals were identified as multilayer reflectors, diffraction gratings, liquid crystals, light scattering structures, and natural photonic crystals.

Despite soft tissues rarely fossilize whilst maintaining the full original information, different eye structures were found in fossils, adding pieces to the evolution of the human eye puzzle.

8.2.2 Structure of Eyes

The human eye can be divided into two main chambers, namely the anterior and the posterior segments. The anterior chamber hosts cornea, iris and lens. Vitreous, retina, choroid, optic nerve, and sclera are located in the posterior chamber.

The cornea acts as a protection for the front-eye side, and it focuses light into the retina.

The sclera is the outer white shell, connected to the cornea via the limbus. The iris is a pigmented circular structure surrounding the pupil, which is capable to adjust its dilation together with the sphincter muscles to regulate the amount of light entering the eye.

The ciliary body produces the aqueous humor, located between lens and cornea, with *immunological* and nourishment functions, which drains from the posterior to the anterior chamber via the pupil, maintaining an intraocular pressure (IOP) of 12~22 mmHg in healthy conditions.

The most relevant eye structures in the framework of this chapter are cornea and sclera. All contact lenses are used in direct contact to the cornea and/or the sclera. The human vision process starts in the eye, where the optical input is received. Light enters the eye through cornea, pupil and lens. Photons reaching the inner retina are converted into electrical signals by rods and cones, *photoreceptive cells* that respond to different intensities and wavelengths of light. Intrinsically photosensitive retinal ganglion cells project to the lateral geniculate nucleus, where the electrical signals travel to three sites of the visual cortex.

Tears are biofluids that may reflect ocular and systemic physiological health. The tear fluid nourishes the ocular surface tissues, and flushes away the waste products of corneal *metabolism*.

Tears can be divided in three main layers.
- The outer lipid layer: secreted by the *meibomian glands*.
- The aqueous layer: secreted by the *lacrimal glands*.
- The mucin layer: produced by the *conjunctival globet cells*.

The tear fluid is composed of a mixture of lipids, electrolytes, proteins, peptides, glucose and amino-acids.

Tear lipids are involved in anti-inflammatory processes. They maintain tear film stability. They reduce the surface free energy, act as a barrier to the aqueous layer, and control water evaporation from the ocular surface.

8.3 PROPERTIES OF CONTACT LENS MATERIALS

Ideal properties for contact lens material are *durability*, *stability,* clarity of vision, and the ability to preserve corneal metabolism by allowing a sufficient oxygen flow to the cornea. *Properties* of contact lenses may be grouped in mechanical, optical, and chemical. Contact lenses are also defined and designed considering a range of geometrical properties.

8.3.1 Chemical Properties

Chemical properties with highest significance with regard to contact lens *polymers* are wettability, water content, oxygen permeability, and swell factor. The surface properties of a polymer determines the way it will interact with the tear fluid. In vivo wettability is evaluated by *tear film breakup time* and interferometry tests, and it reflects the ability of the contact lens to keep a stable tear film within the ocular surface. In vitro wettability is assessed by evaluating the contact angle at the solid-liquid-air interface, and measuring the hysteresis, i.e., the difference between advanced and receding contact angle.

$$\text{EWC} = \frac{\text{weight of water in polymer}}{\text{total weight of hydrated polymer}} \times 100$$

The *equilibrium* water content (EWC) of a hydrogel is influenced by environmental conditions, pH, tonicity and temperature. The International Organization for Standardization (ISO) defines the regulatory standards for EWC measurements in contact lens hydrogels. Both thermogravimetry and back-calculation by refractive index measurements are considered valid techniques for EWC assessment.

The oxygen permeability is indicated as *Dk*, where *D* is the *diffusivity* and *k* is the *solubility* of the material. *Dk* is an intrinsic characteristic of a contact lens to transmit oxygen to the cornea from the atmosphere. Hydrogels transport oxygen via the water channels and their oxygen permeability is closely related to temperature and EWC, according to the following equation.

$$Dk = 1.67 e^{0.0397 \text{EWC}}$$

The amount of oxygen transported from the anterior to the posterior surface $O_{2, A \to P}$ of a lens can be calculated dividing the oxygen permeability *Dk* by the lens thickness(*t*).

$$O_{2, A \to P} = \frac{Dk}{t}$$

8.3.2 Mechanical Properties

The mechanical properties of contact lenses determine their comfort, visual performance, fitting methods, and durability. Soft lenses are obtained with wettable polymers, and their properties change with *water content*. Mechanical testing involves applying a stress (compression, tensile or shear) and observing the resulting strain. Contact lens polymers are mechanically characterized by their stress-strain curve, and their Young's modulus is defined by the formula $E = \sigma \times \varepsilon^{-1}$, where σ is the applied stress, and ε is the corresponding strain. The modulus of rigid lens materials amounts to 10 GPa, whereas hydrated soft lenses have modulus of 0.2~1.5 MPa. The increased content of siloxy-methacrylates in RGP materials confers them a higher oxygen permeability, but it reduces their dimensional stability.

8.3.3 Optical Properties

Optical properties of contact lenses play a crucial role in providing a good visual performance. The most important optical parameters of a contact lens are optical transparency and refractive index of the polymer. Hydrogels have a light *transmission* > 90%. Sometimes microphase separation of water occurs, negatively affecting hydrogels transparency by creating zones with different refractive indexes. Ideally, the refractive index of a contact lens matches the one of the cornea (1.37). The refractive index is measured using an Abbé refractometer. Fluorosilicone acrylate lenses have a refractive index of 1.42~1.46, and silicone acrylates have a refractive index above 1.460. The refractive index of PMMA is 1.49. Commercial contact lenses with higher refractive indexes (1.51~1.54) are advantageous in a spheric multifocal designs.

8.4 CONTACT LENS MANUFACTURE

Contact lenses are manufactured by shaping a plastic material into specific curvatures, namely the central anterior curve (CAC) and the central posterior curve (CPC). Contact lenses may be manufactured by either *molding* or *lathe cutting*. Molding is an additive process that consists on curing a solution inside a lens-shaped mold, and it is used for mass-production in general prescriptions. Lathe cutting is a subtractive process where a blank of material is modelled to the desired shape for individual prescriptions.

8.4.1 Molding

The molding process is primarily dedicated to soft lenses fabrication. It can be done by spin-casting, compression, or injection. The first soft lenses were obtained by spin casting. Compression molding was used in the past for PMMA lenses fabrication, but it has now fallen out of fashion. Nowadays, individually packaged, disposable soft contact lenses are mass-produced by spin casting (*Figure 8-2 a*) and injection molding (*Figure 8-2 b*). The contact lens solution is spun at a controlled speed inside a mold, resulting in the liquid being uniformly spread all over the mold, under UV curing. The resulting lens is peeled off, edged and hydrated. Lenses are then autoclaved and packaged. The injection molding process is equivalent to spin casting, but the lens is shaped by using a two-pieces mold. In injection molding, the molten plastic is injected into the mold under pressure and cured under UV irradiation. The lens is peeled off, cooled, and finished on a lathe. Contact lenses are finally softened by hydration prior to undergoing quality assurance tests.

8.4.2 Lathe Cutting

Lathe cutting is primarily adopted in *customized* rigid lenses production, but soft lenses can also be fabricated by lathe cutting in a similar manner. The fabrication of rigid lenses by lathe cutting is illustrated in Figure 8-2 c.

8.5 NOMENCLATURE FOR CONTACT LENS

Contact lens is an artificial device whose front surface substitutes the anterior surface of the cornea. Therefore, in addition to correction of refractive error, the irregularities of the front surface of cornea can also be corrected by the contact lenses. The parts, curves, and nomenclature for contact lens are as follows.

8.5.1 Diameters of the Lens
- *Overall diameter (OD)* of the lens is the linear measurement of the greatest distance across the physical boundaries of lens. It is expressed in millimetres. (It should not be confused as being twice the radius of curvature.)
- *Optic zone diameter (OZ)* is the dimension of the central optic zone of lens which is meant to focus rays on retina.

8.5.2 Curves of the Lens
- *Base curve (BC)* or central posterior curve (CPC) is a curve on the back surface of the lens to fit the front surface of cornea.
- *Peripheral curves*. These are concentric to base curve and include intermediate posterior curve (IPC) and peripheral posterior curve (PPC). These are meant to serve as reservoir of tears and to form a ski for lens movements.
- Central anterior curve (CAC) or front curve (FC) is the curve on the anterior surface of the optical zone of the lens. Its curvature determines the power of contact lens.
- Peripheral anterior curve (PAC) is a slope on the periphery of anterior surface which goes up to the edge.
- Intermediate anterior curve (IAC) is fabricated only in the high power minus and plus lenses. It lies between the CAC and PAC.

8.5.3 Edge of the Lens
- It is the polished and blended union of the peripheral posterior and anterior curves of the lens.

8.5.4 Power of the Lens
- It is measured in terms of posterior vertex power in dioptres.

8.5.5 Thickness of the Lens
- It is usually measured in the centre of the lens and varies depending upon the posterior vertex power of the lens.

8.5.6 Tint
- It is the colour of the lens.

8.6 TYPES OF CONTACT LENS

Contact lenses interact with the ocular surface via the tear film, the corneal epithelium, and the conjunctival epithelium. A contact lens must allow sufficient oxygen flow to maintain aerobic metabolism, corneal *homeostasis*, and tear film stability. Contact lenses are classified in many different ways: by their primary function, material, wear schedule (how long a lens can be worn), and replacement schedule (how long before a lens needs to be discarded).

Depending upon the nature of the material used in their manufacturing, the contact lenses can be divided into the following three types: a. hard lenses; b. rigid gas permeable lenses; c. soft contact lenses.

8.6.1 Hard Lenses

Hard lenses are used to address astigmatism and corneal *irregularities* with a variety of designs, including front-toric, back-toric, and bi-toric. The first hard lenses were made of glass, now they are manufactured from PMMA (polymethyl methacrylate). The PMMA has a high optical quality, stability and is light in weight, non-toxic, durable and cheap. However, PMMA shows substantial limitations in terms of corneal respiration, which increases the risk of undergoing ocular *complications*. The hard corneal lenses have a diameter of 8.5~10 mm. Presently these are not used commonly.

Disadvantages of PMMA hard contact lenses:
- PMMA is practically impermeable to O_2 thus restricting the *tolerance*.
- Being hard, it can cause corneal *abrasions*.
- Being *hydrophobic* in nature, resists *wetting* but a stable tear film can be formed over it.

Note: PMMA contact lenses are sparingly used in clinical practice because of poor patient acceptance.

8.6.2 Rigid Gas Permeable Lenses (RGP)
8.6.2.1 Rigid gas permeable lenses (RGP)

Rigid gas permeable (RGP) lenses (*Figure 8-4 a*) are made up of materials which are permeable to oxygen. Basically these are also hard, but somehow due to their O_2 permeability they have become popular by the name of semi-soft lenses. Gas permeable lenses are commonly manufactured from *copolymer* of PMMA and silicone containing *vinyl monomer*. Cellulose acetate butyrate (CAB), a class of *thermoplastic* material derived from special grade wood cellulose has also been used, but is not popular. Siloxy-methacrylate-based materials with enhanced wettability laid the foundations to the development of Boston RPG materials. Menicon is credited with introducing the first contact lenses with hyperoxygen transmissibility (Dk=175), composed of tris (trimethyl-siloxy) silyl styrene and fluoromethacrylate. As of 2019, Menicon Z contact lenses are the only rigid lenses that received FDA approval for 30 days of *continuous wear*.

Rigid lenses were initially fabricated as corneal lenses or scleral lenses, with diameters ranging from 7.0 to 12.0 mm, and above 18.0 mm, respectively. Over the past decade, therapeutics drove the market toward manufacturing rigid lenses with intermediate dimensions. Nowadays, rigid lenses are used in the form of corneoscleral lenses, with diameters ranging from 12.0 to 15.0 mm, and mini-scleral lenses, with diameters of 15.0 to 18.0 mm.

8.6.2.2 Orthokeratology

Orthokeratology (also referred to as Ortho-K), a special type of contact lens that uses rigid materials, ensuring the best oxygen transmission rate, has become increasingly popular for controlling myopic progression (*Figure 8-4 b*). The concept of orthokeratology (OK) was first introduced in the 1950s by Wesley and Jessen as spectacle blur, a phenomenon describing corneal reshaping after wearing hard contact lenses. For its material was poor at oxygen permeation, making long-term wearing infeasible, orthokeratology was more of a novelty back then. In the 1970s, rigid gas permeable lenses improved comfort and safety by allowing more oxygen permeability. However, the lenses still remained incapable of effectively correcting myopia until the first reverse geometry lens designed by Richard Wlodyga introduced in 1989, which improved lens centration and myopia correction from −1 diopters (D) to −1.7 D. Up to the present, improvement of orthokeratology mainly involves using higher Dk lens material, different reverse geometry lens designs, and advances in *corneal topography*.

By the reverse geometry design of orthokeratology lens, the lens molds the cornea of a myopic eye into plateau shape. These orthokeratology lenses have much flatter central base curve than the secondary curve, thus create positive pushing pressure against the central cornea and negative pulling pressure against the mid-peripheral cornea, *redistributing* the epithelial cells to the mid-periphery while flattening the central cornea via a thinning of the epithelial layer. Through plateau-shaped cornea, light would be refracted simultaneously onto the mid-peripheral retina and macula, leaving the peripheral retina with relative myopic defocus. Hyperopic peripheral defocus on the contrary, often found in myopic children, is believed to encourage eye growth. Manipulation of peripheral defocus toward myopia is hypothesized to stabilize eye growth and reduce myopia progression.

Nowadays, overnight orthokeratology is becoming more and more popular especially in the Asia-Pacific region to control the progression of myopia in young children. Overnight orthokeratology is worn during sleep to *reshape* the front surface of the cornea for the purpose of temporary reduction of refractive errors. Reduction of refractive error in myopia was thought to be the result of central corneal flattening, thickening of the midperipheral cornea, thinning of the central corneal epithelium, and peripheral vision myopic shift. The patients, especially young myopes with low and moderate myopia, will own useful vision during waking hours through wearing this reverse geometry-designed lenses during sleep. The reverse geometry lenses reshape the cornea intentionally by positive pressure in the center of cornea, as well as negative pressure in the midperiphery to reduce or eliminate refractive error temporarily. It makes the central cornea flattening to correct axial myopia and midperipheral cornea steepening to reduce relative peripheral hyperopia. Plenty of studies have demonstrated that wearing overnight orthokeratology can slow the progression of myopia effectively and safely.

8.6.2.3 Scleral lenses

According to the official document adopted by the Scleral Lens Education Society (SLS), scleral lenses should be defined as follows: a lens fitted to vault over the entire cornea, including the limbus, and to land on conjunctiva overlying the sclera (*Figure 8-3*). Simply put, if a lens rests completely on the cornea, it is called a corneal lens. A lens that partly rests on the cornea (centrally or peripherally), and partly on the sclera is called a corneo-scleral lens. A lens that rests entirely on the sclera, is a scleral lens no matter how large that lens is.

With increasing interest of clinicians and manufacturers, scleral lenses have become "mainstream" in specialty contact lens practice to benefit patients. Scleral lenses are presently manufactured in highly oxygen permeable rigid gas permeable materials. Current materials allow high levels of oxygen to pass through the lens compared to early PMMA lenses. Therefore, corneal *edema* is not commonly reported in scleral lenses wear.

Scleral lenses are usually not a first option, but are typically prescribed when other lenses do not provide adequate visual acuity or are not well tolerated. The motivation for fitting scleral lenses is typically divided into vision improvement, ocular surface protection and support, and a segment that includes fitting scleral lenses for sports and *cosmetic* purposes. While some studies report only on the application of these lenses in severe ocular surface disease for surface protection, others include only the application for corneal irregularities. Recent studies have reported a wider scope of ocular conditions including irregularity of the ocular surface, such as in *keratoconus*, post surgical ectasia or post *keratoplasty* and so on.

8.6.3 Soft Lenses

Soft lenses are made of hydrogels, i.e. water-containing polymers, which allow better comfort and higher flexibility than rigid lenses (*Figure 8-4 c*). Soft lenses are 2~3 mm larger than the cornea, with a diameter of 14.5 mm. They are produced solely in the form of corneal lenses, and they lay on the cornea. Every contact lens is a barrier to oxygen transportation into the eye and can induce hypoxia, which is a cause of clinical problems, such as corneal edema, corneal *neovascularization*, corneal *acidosis*, loss of corneal transparency, *epithelial keratitis*, and *endothelial* polymegathism.

Soft lens materials have been developed to be more *biocompatible*, especially with respect to increased oxygen permeability (*Dk*). Because of the relatively low *Dk* of traditional hydrogel lenses, the minimum oxygen requirement of the cornea is not met under closed eyelid conditions. To counteract the potential clinical problems induced by low *Dk* of conventional hydrogel lens during overnight wear, new types of hydrogel lens materials containing organosilicone moieties in their polymers have been developed. Silicone hydrogels were first introduced in 1998. *Silicone hydrogel lenses* exhibited increased water content and lower modulus, have about 5~10 times the *Dk* of traditional hydrogel materials, resulting in a lower incidence of *papillary conjunctivitis* associated to contact lens wear.

- Advantages: Being soft and oxygen permeable, they are most comfortable and so well tolerated.
- Disadvantages: Include problem of wettability, *proteinaceous deposits,* getting cracked, limited life, inferior optical quality, more chances of corneal infections and cannot correct astigmatism of more than 2 D.

Note: In clinical practice soft lenses are most frequently prescribed.

Depending upon the functions, the contact lenses can be divided into the following three types: corrective contact lenses, cosmetic contact lenses, therapeutic contact lenses.

8.6.4 Corrective Contact Lenses

A *corrective contact lens* is designed to improve vision. In many people, there is a mismatch between the refractive power of the eye and the length of the eye, leading to a refraction error. A contact lens neutralizes this mismatch and allows for correct focusing of light onto the retina. Conditions correctable with contact lenses include myopia (near or short sightedness), hypermetropia (far or long sightedness), astigmatism and presbyopia. Contact wearers must usually take their contact lenses out every night or every few days, depending on the brand and style of the contact. Recently, there has been renewed interest in orthokeratology, the correction of myopia by deliberate overnight flattening of the cornea, leaving the eye without contact lens or eyeglasses correction during the day.

For those with certain *color deficiencies*, a red-*tinted* ChromaGen contact lens may be used. Although the lens does not restore normal color vision, it allows some *colorblind* individuals to distinguish colors better. ChromaGen lenses have been used and these have been shown to have some limitations with vision at night although otherwise producing significant improvements in color vision. An earlier study showed very significant improvements in color vision and patient satisfaction. Later work that used these ChromaGen lenses with *dyslexics* in a randomised, double-blind, placebo controlled trial showed highly significant improvements in reading ability over reading without the lenses.

8.6.5 Cosmetic Contact Lenses

A *cosmetic contact lens* is designed to change the appearance of the eye. These lenses may also correct the vision, but some blurring or obstruction of vision may occur as a result of the color or design. In the USA, the FDA frequently calls non-corrective cosmetic contact lenses decorative contact lenses. These types of lenses tend to cause mild *irritation* on *insertion*, but after the eyes become accustomed, tend to cause no long term damage. Though it is advised that these lenses not be worn too much, research has shown them to have no direct link to any forms of eye degradation. Although many brands of contact lenses are lightly tinted to make them easier to handle, cosmetic lenses worn to change the color of the eye are far less common.

8.6.6 Therapeutic Contact Lenses

Soft lenses are often used in the treatment and management of non-refractive disorders of the eye. A *bandage contact lens* protects an injured or diseased cornea from the constant rubbing of blinking eyelids, thereby allowing it to heal. They are used in the treatment of conditions including *bullous keratopathy*, *dry eyes*, corneal *ulcers* and *erosion*, keratitis, corneal edema, *descemetocele*, Mooren's ulcer, anterior corneal *dystrophy*, and neurotrophic *keratoconjunctivitis*. Contact lenses that deliver drugs to the eye have also been developed.

8.6.7 Some Other Types

The various soft contact lenses available are often categorized by their wear time, replacement schedule or design.

8.6.7.1 By wear time

A *daily wear* contact lens is designed to be removed prior to sleeping. An *extended wear (EW)* contact lens is designed for continuous overnight wear, typically for 6 or more consecutive nights. Newer materials, such as silicone hydrogels, allow for even longer wear periods of up to 30 consecutive nights; these longer-wear lenses are often referred to as *continuous wear (CW)*. Generally, extended wear lenses are *discarded* after the specified length of time. These are increasing in popularity, due to their obvious convenience. Extended- and continuous-wear contact lenses can be worn for such long periods of time because of their high oxygen permeability (typically 5~6 times greater than conventional soft lenses), which allows the eye to remain healthy.

Extended lens wearers may have an increased risk for corneal infections and corneal ulcers, primarily due to poor care and cleaning of the lenses, tear film instability, and *bacterial stagnation*. Corneal neovascularization has historically also been a common complication of extended lens wear, though this does not appear to be a problem with silicone hydrogel extended wear. The most common complication of extended lens use is conjunctivitis, usually *allergic* or *giant papillary conjunctivitis (GPC)*, sometimes associated with a poorly fitting contact lens.

8.6.7.2 By replacement schedule

The shortest replacement schedule is single use (*daily disposable*) lenses, which are disposed of each night. Shorter replacement cycle lenses are commonly thinner and lighter, due to lower requirements for durability against wear and tear, and may be the most comfortable. These may be best for patients with ocular allergies or other conditions, because it limits deposits of *antigens* and *protein*. More commonly, contact lenses are prescribed to be disposed of on a two-week or monthly basis. Quarterly or annual lenses, which used to be very common, have lost favor because a more frequent disposal schedule allows for thinner lenses and limits deposits. Rigid gas permeable lenses are very durable and may last for several years without the need for replacement.

8.6.7.3 By design

A spherical contact lens is one in which both the inner and outer optical surfaces are portions of a sphere. A toric lens is one in which either or both of the optical surfaces have the effect of a cylindrical lens, usually in combination with the effect of a spherical lens. Myopic and hypermetropic people who also have astigmatism and who have been told they are not suitable for regular contact lenses may be able to use toric lenses. If one eye has astigmatism and the other does not, the patient may be told to use a spherical lens in one eye and a toric lens in the other.

Like eyeglasses, contact lenses can have one (single vision) or more (multifocal) focal points.

Multifocal contact lenses (e.g. bifocals or progressives) are comparable to spectacles with bifocals or progressive lenses because they have multiple focal points. Multifocal contact lenses are typically designed for constant viewing through the center of the lens, but some designs do incorporate a shift in lens position to view through the reading power (similar to bifocal glasses). However, multifocal contact lenses, which use *simultaneous* imaging, often cause visual disturbances, such as *ghosting* and *haloes*, because the optical zones for intermediate- and near-distance focusing are positioned over the pupil. These disturbances can occur at any distance and are often exacerbated in *low-contrast* or low-illumination conditions. Such effects range from mild to severe and have been demonstrated to be associated with pupil size, lens *decentration*, lens design, and inherent spherical aberration. Many currently used multifocal contact lenses are designed to satisfy the complex visual requirements of patients with presbyopia while minimizing the negative effects.

Monovision is the use of single-vision lenses (one focal point per lens) to focus an eye (typically the dominant one) for distance vision and the other for near work. The brain then learns to use this setup to see clearly at all distances. A technique called modified monovision uses multifocal lenses and also specializes one eye for distance and the other for near, thus gaining the benefits of both systems. Alternatively, a person may simply wear reading glasses over their distance contact lenses. Care is advised for persons with a previous history of strabismus and those with significant phorias, who are at risk of eye *misalignment* under monovision.

8.7 THE APPLICATION OF CONTACT LENSES

8.7.1 Advantages of Contact Lenses over Spectacles
- Irregular corneal astigmatism which is not possible to correct with glasses can be corrected with contact lenses.
- Contact lenses provide normal field of vision.
- Aberrations associated with spectacles (such as peripheral aberrations and prismatic distortions) are eliminated.
- Binocular vision can be retained in high anisometropia (e.g. unilateral aphakia) owing to less magnification of the retinal image.
- Rain and fog do not condense upon contact lenses as they do on spectacles.
- Cosmetically more acceptable especially by females and all patients with thick glasses in high refractive errors.

8.7.2 Contraindications for Contact Lens Use
- Mental incompetence, and poor motivation.
- *Chronic dacryocystitis*.
- Chronic *blepharitis* and *recurrent* styes.
- Chronic conjunctivitis.
- Dry-eye syndromes.
- Corneal dystrophies and degenerations.
- Recurrent diseases like *episcleritis*, *scleritis* and *iridocyclitis*.

8.7.3 Indications of Contact Lens Use
Optical indications include anisometropia, unilateral aphakia, high myopia, keratoconus and irregular astigmatism. Optically they can be used by every patient having refractive error for cosmetic purposes.

8.7.3.1 Therapeutic indications
- Corneal diseases, e.g. non-healing corneal ulcers, bullous keratopathy, filamentary keratitis and recurrent corneal erosion syndrome.
- Diseases of iris such as *aniridia*, *coloboma* and albinism to avoid glare.
- In glaucoma as vehicle for drug delivery.
- In amblyopia, opaque contact lenses are used for occlusion.
- Bandage soft contact lenses are used following keratoplasty and in microcorneal *perforation*.

8.7.3.2 Preventive indications
- Prevention of symblepharon and restoration of fornices in chemical burns.

- Exposure keratitis.
- Trichiasis.

8.7.3.3 Diagnostic indications
- Gonioscopy.
- Electroretinography.
- Examination of fundus in the presence of irregular corneal astigmatism.
- Fundus photography.
- Goldmann's 3 mirror examination.

8.7.3.4 Operative indications
- Goniotomy operation for *congenital glaucoma*.
- *Vitrectomy*.
- Endocular photocoagulation.

8.7.3.5 Cosmetic indications
- Unsightly corneal scars (colour contact lenses).
- Ptosis (haptic contact lens).
- Cosmetic scleral lenses in phthisis bulbi.

8.7.3.6 Occupational indications
- Sportsmen.
- Pilots.
- Actors.

Chapter 9
Diseases of the Cornea

ANATOMY AND PHYSIOLOGY OF THE CORNEA
GENERAL INTRODUCTION TO KERATITIS
HERPES SIMPLEX KERATITIS (HSK)
HERPES ZOSTER OPHTHALMICUS (HZO)
BACTERIAL CORNEA ULCER
ACANTHAMOEBA KERATITIS (AK)
EXPOSURE KERATITIS
KERATOCONUS

9.1 ANATOMY AND PHYSIOLOGY OF THE CORNEA

The cornea forms anterior one-sixth of the outer fibrous coat of the eyeball, and it is an avascular, transparent, watch-glass like structure. The cornea is supplied by anterior ciliary nerves which are branches of ophthalmic division of the 5th cranial nerve. The two primary physiological functions of cornea are:
- to act as a major refractive medium.
- to protect the intraocular contents.

The cornea is divided into five layers from front to back :
- Epithelium.
- Bowman's membrane.
- Stroma.
- Descemet's membrane (posterior elastic lamina).
- Endothelium.

9.2 GENERAL INTRODUCTION TO KERATITIS

Any cause of corneal tissue inflammation is collectively referred to as keratitis. Common symptoms of keratitis are red eye, foreign body sensation, eye pain, sensitivity to light, watery eyes, blurry vision, decrease in vision. Keratitis may be mild, moderate, or severe, and can be associated with inflammation of other regions of the eye. It may also involve one eye (unilateral) or both eyes (bilateral).

Keratitis may or may not be associated with an infection. Noninfectious keratitis can be caused by a relatively minor injury, by overexposure to ultraviolet light, by weak immunity, by wearing contact lenses too long or by a foreign body in the eye. Treatment of noninfectious keratitis varies depending on the severity. For example, artificial tears may be the only treatment for mild discomfort caused by a corneal scratch. However, if keratitis causes significant tearing and pain, topical eye medication may be required. Infectious keratitis can be caused by bacteria, viruses, fungi or parasites. Treatment of infectious keratitis varies, depending on the cause of the infection.

9.3 HERPES SIMPLEX KERATITIS (HSK)

Herpetic eye disease is the most prevalent infectious cause of corneal blindness in developed countries. Age, geographic location, and socioeconomic status appear to affect the prevalence of disease. HSK is caused by recurrent infection of the cornea (the clear dome that covers the colored part of the eye), which is caused by HSV (Herpes Simplex Virus). The infection usually heals without damage the eye, but more severe infection can lead to scarring of the cornea or blindness. It can easily progress to corneal perforation or blindness if left unchecked. Symptoms of HSK include eye pain, eye redness, blurry vision, sensitivity to light, watery discharge. HSV is enveloped and has a linear double-stranded DNA genome. Its only natural host is human. Basically HSV is epitheliotropic but may become neurotropic. According to different clinical and immunological properties, there are two types of HSV, each affecting different regions of the body.

- Type 1: HSV-I typically causes infection above the waist, which is acquired by kissing or coming in close contact with a patient suffering from herpes labialis. HSV-I is the type of HSV that causes cold sores on the mouth. It is also the most common cause of corneal infections. Seroprevalence of HSV-I is over 50% in the US while more than 75% in Germany.
- Type 2: HSV-II typically causes infection below the waist (herpes genitalis). It has also been reported to cause ocular lesions. It may get transmitted to the eye through infected secretions, either venereally or at birth.

Ocular involvement by HSV comes in two forms, primary and recurrent infection:
- Primary infection: The primary infection (the first attack) involves a non-immune

person. Primary infection may occur at any point in life. It typically occurs in children between 6 months and 5 years of age and in teenagers. In addition, HSV transmission facilitation occurs in conditions of crowding and poor hygiene. Patients may suffer from the skin lesions, acute follicular conjunctivitis, cornea lesion (fine epithelial punctate keratitis, coarse epithelial punctate keratitis, dendritic ulcer, etc.)

- Recurrent infection: Primary infection may become latent, the virus which lies dormant in the trigeminal ganglion, periodically reactivates and causes recurrent infection. Predisposing stress stimuli which trigger an attack of herpetic keratitis include sunlight, trauma, heat, menstruation, stress, trigeminal nerve manipulation, infectious disease and immunocompromised states. Patients may suffer from the active epithelial keratitis (punctate epithelial keratitis, dendritic ulcer, geographical ulcer), stromal keratitis (disciform keratitis, diffuse stromal necrotic keratitis), trophic keratitis (meta-herpetic), herpetic iridocyclitis, etc.

9.4 HERPES ZOSTER OPHTHALMICUS(HZO)

Herpes Zosters Ophthalmicus (HZO), is a viral disease characterized by a unilateral painful skin rash in one or more dermatome distributions of the fifth cranial nerve (trigeminal nerve), shared by the eye and ocular adnexa. It accounts for about 10% of all cases of Herpes Zoster(HZ), which is commonly known as shingles.

HZ is caused by the varicella-zoster virus (VZV) (a DNA virus). The virulence of the VZV and the immune status of the host are the main factors leading to the occurence of HZO. Immune system status plays a role, and patients treated with immunosuppressive drugs have a significantly increased risk of developing HZ. Immunocompromised patients are more likely to have a long-term illness, are more likely to relapse and are more likely to develop myelitis and vascular disease. People with HIV have a greater risk of getting HZ than people without HIV. The infection is acquired in childhood, which manifests as chickenpox and the child develops immunity. Anyone who has had chickenpox, even in subclinical form, is at risk for developing HZ. The virus then lies dormant in the sensory ganglion of the fifth cranial nerve. It is thought that the virus reactivates, replicates and spreads down along one or more branches of the ophthalmic division of the fifth cranial nerve, usually occurring in older people with compromised cellular immunity (it can actually occur at any age). The incidence and severity of HZ increases with age, with patients over 60 years of age at highest risk.

Clinical features of HZO are as follows:

① Signs: Erythematous skin lesions with macules, papules, vesicles, pustules, and crusting lesions in the distribution of the trigeminal nerve, in which frontal nerve is more frequently affected than the lacrimal and nasociliary nerves. Lesions of herpes zoster are strictly limited to one side of the midline of head. Hutchinson's sign is defined as skin lesions at the tip, side, or root of the nose, which is a strong predictor of ocular inflammation and corneal denervation, especially if both branches of the nasociliary nerve are involved. However, the Hutchinson's rule is useful but not infallible. HZO iritis is frequently associated with high intraocular pressure.

② Symptoms: Many cases of HZO exhibit a prodromal period of fever, malaise, headache, and eye pain prior to the eruption of the skin rash. Dermatome distribution pain and rash with associated ocular findings strongly suggest HZO. Pain in the distribution of the trigeminal nerve may be severe. Corneal epithelial defects, decreased corneal sensation, and ocular inflammation in any of the layers of the eye also correlate with the diagnosis.

The most important step of defensing against HZO is vaccination. An effective vaccine has been approved in the United States, Europe, and China. However, HZ remains common worldwide, in part because of lack of knowledge of the vaccine, as well as limited access to and shortages of the vaccine. This vaccine is recommended for immunocompetent adults ≥ 50 years, regardless of whether they have had HZ or been given the older, live-attenuated vaccine. The standard treatment for HZ is antiviral medication (e.g. acyclovir, famciclovir, valacyclovir), preferably initiated within 72 hours of rash onset. Patients with uveitis or keratitis require topical corticosteroids (e.g. prednisolone acetate). Intraocular pressure must be monitored and treated if it rises significantly above normal values. In addition, adjuvant therapy is used for HZO. Analgesics or steroids are given to reduce pain. If blinking is impaired, lubricating and antibiotic ophthalmic ointments may be used.

9.5 BACTERIAL CORNEA ULCER

The cornea is the "window" of the eye. A corneal ulcer is an open sore on the cornea, which can lead to permanent damage, even blindness if it's not treated, so it's considered to be a medical emergency. Like ulcers elsewhere in the body, corneal ulcers are complete destruction of the epithelial cell layer, accompanied by an inflammatory response. Unlike the rest of the body, the cornea is dehydrated and avascular, both of which contribute to its clarity and transparency. However, the avascular nature of the cornea presents a challenge for the body to resist infection because the immune system is impaired. Thus, infection is the leading cause of corneal ulcer. Infective corneal ulcers can occur in the presence of impaired ocular defense mechanisms, predisposing ocular diseases, compromised host immunity, or virulent pathogens. Infective causes of corneal ulcers include bacterial infections, viral infections, fungal infections, and parasitic infections. Non-infective causes can also lead to corneal ulcers, including eyelid closure problems, autoimmune diseases, vitamin A deficiency, severe dry eyes, etc.

Bacterial corneal ulcers can develop in healthy patients due to long-term contact lens use, but burned patients are particularly at risk due to factors such as loss of eyelid function, ocular surface exposure, local contamination, and disrupted host immunity. Pathogens include Acinetobacter spp., Staphylococcus spp., Pseudomonas spp., etc. In bacterial infections, the outcome depends on the virulence of the pathogen as well as the host's response. Symptoms of a bacterial corneal ulcer include pain and foreign body sensation, tearing, photophobia, blurry vision, and redness. There are a number of manifestations that clinicians can detect through slit-lamp observations, such as the swollen eyelids, marked blepharospasm, hypopyon, chemosis, conjunctival hyperaemia and/or ciliary congestion, stromal oedema, etc. Corneal ulcer usually starts as an epithelial defect associated with greyish-white circumscribed infiltrate (seen in early stage), followed by expansion of the epithelial defect and infiltration. Central corneal ulcers are usually more severe than periphery corneal ulcers.

Bacterial corneal ulcers are a vision threatening disease that urgently needs to be treated by identifying and eradicating the pathogenic bacteria. Delayed treatment may result in corneal perforation, endophthalmitis and/or permanent corneal scarring and visual impairment.

9.6 ACANTHAMOEBA KERATITIS (AK)

The incidence of acanthamoeba keratitis has been rising over the past several decades. Free-living acanthamoeba species are the causative agents of a severe vision-threatening corneal infection called acanthamoeba keratitis. It can be found in soil, fresh water, well water, sea water, sewage and air, and exists in two forms, an active trophozoite or a dormant cyst. AK is hard to diagnose, so AK should be considered in all contact lens wearers and in any case of corneal trauma with exposure to soil or contaminated water. To diagnose it, all patients with suspected eye infections need a detailed medical history, and the sampling and investigation of the correct material is very important. Only if amoebae are detected in corneal scrapings or in corneal biopsies a reliable diagnosis can be made. The sooner the disease is diagnosed, the better the outcome.

AK results from direct corneal contact with any material or water contaminated with the organism. There are 4 common situations:
- Contact lens wearers (the leading risk factor of AK).
- People suffered from mild trauma associated with contaminated vegetable matter, salt water diving, wind blown contaminant and hot tub use.
- Opportunistic infection in patients with herpetic keratitis, bacterial keratitis, bullous keratopathy and neuroparalytic keratitis.
- Non-contact lens wearers, especially individuals with regular ocular exposure to dust, soil, or contaminated water.

Acanthamoeba keratitis is usually unilateral but may occur in both eyes. Patients often complain about the massive pain (out of proportion to the degree of inflammation), decreased vision, eye redness, foreign body sensation, photophobia, tearing, and discharge. Symptoms can range from mild to severe. Acanthamoeba keratitis worsens gradually over several months, with brief periods of remission. There are marked changes in presentation that make diagnosis difficult. In the early stage, findings on slit-lamp examination including an epitheliopathy with punctuate keratopathy, epithelial or subepithelial infiltrates, pseudodendrites, and perineural infiltrates. In the late stage, findings on the slit-lamp examination including "ring-like" stromal infiltrate, radial keratoneuritis, satellite lesions, ulceration, abscess formation, anterior uveitis with hypopyon, and epithelial defects.

The treatment of AK is usually unsatisfactory. Acanthamoeba trophozoites are relatively sensitive to a variety of medications, including antibiotics, antiseptics, antifungals, and antiprotozoals. However, Acanthamoeba cysts are resistant to most of the listed treatments, thereby allowing for prolonged infection.

9.7 EXPOSURE KERATITIS

Normally, the cornea is covered by the eyelids during sleep and kept moist by blinking when awake. If disease process causes inadequate eyelid closure, the condition of exposure keratopathy (keratitis lagophthalmos) develops. Many factors that produce lagophthalmos may lead to exposure keratitis: neurogenic diseases such as Bell's palsy, acoustic neuroma; proptosis due to thyroid orbitopathy or other orbital diseases; eyelid dysfunction from restrictive eyelid diseases or previous blepharoplasty; inattentive mental states such as in comatose patients or nocturnal exposure.

Patients with exposure keratitis may have some symptoms, including foreign body sensation, itching, burning and conjunctival injection, blurry vision, pain and photophobia. Clinicians can find the signs on the cornea through slit-lamp examination. Superficial punctate epithelial staining involves inferior third of the cornea usually. If timely treatments are not taken, patients may progress to large area of epithelial defect and complicated with corneal infiltrates, ulceration, perforation or endophthalmitis.

The principle of treatment is always to target the underlying causes. To make sure the cornea is moist, there are several ways to do this, such as using the nonpreserved topical drops during the day and lubricating ointment at bedtime. Lid taping and moisture chamber glasses are also useful. Moisture chamber glasses surround, enclose the eyes and keep out the air, so it takes longer for patient's tears to dry out. Antibiotic is also essential for epithelial corneal defects.

9.8 KERATOCONUS

Keratoconus occurs when collagen protein fibers in the eye become weak and thin, thus the cornea thins and gradually bulges outward into a cone shape. The ability to focus light diminishes, causing vision loss. Keratoconus is a non-inflammatory ectatic condition of cornea in its axial part. However, more recently it has been associated with ocular inflammation. Keratoconus usually affects both eyes, though it often affects one eye more than the other. It generally begins to affect people between the ages of 10 and 25. The condition may progress slowly for 10 years or longer. Keratoconus causes blurry vision and may cause sensitivity to light and glare. The etiopathogenesis of keratoconus is still not clear. A family history of keratoconus, eye rubbing, eczema, asthma, and allergy are risk factors for developing keratoconus. Detecting keratoconus in its earliest stages remains a challenge. Corneal topography is the primary diagnostic tool for keratoconus detection. Corneal pachymetry and higher order aberration data are now commonly used.

For patients with keratoconus, the symptoms can vary from person to person. The most common signs and symptoms include blurry vision, sensitivity to light, poor night vision, double vision, ghost images (incomplete image), myopia, irregular astigmatism, etc. During the eye examination, we can find the window reflex is distorted, placido disc examination shows irregular circles, and keratometry depicts extreme malalignment of mires. Slit lamp examination may show thinning and ectasia of central cornea, opacity at the apex and Fleischer's ring at the base of cone, and folds in Descemet's and Bowman's membranes. Very fine, vertical, deep stromal striae (Vogt lines) which disappear with external pressure on the globe are unique features. Munson's sign, which means localised bulging of lower lid when patient looks down is positive in late stages. Keratoconus posterior is an extremely rare condition. There is slight cone-like bulging of the posterior surface of the cornea. It is non-progressive.

Depending upon the size and shape of the cone. The keratoconus is of three types.
- Nipple cone: a small size (<5 mm) and steep curvature.
- Oval cone: a medium size (5~6 mm) and ellipsoid in shape.
- Globus cone: a large size (>6 mm) and globe like.

There is no way to completely cure keratoconus. Falling vision may not be corrected by glasses due to irregular astigmatism. In the early stages of keratoconus, patient's vision problems could be corrected with glasses or soft contact lenses. Later, rigid gas permeable contact lenses or other types of lenses could be utilized, such as scleral lenses. If patient's condition progresses to an advanced stage, intacs (intracorneal ring segments) are reported to be useful. At last, keratoplasty (cornea transplant) may be required. If left untreated, keratoconus can lead to permanent vision loss. LASIK eye surgery is not recommended for people with keratoconus because it can worsen the condition.

Chapter 10
Glaucoma

INTRODUCTION
- The Definition of Glaucoma
- Intraocular Pressure and Glaucoma

CLASSIFICATION OF GLAUCOMA
- Primary Glaucoma
- Secondary Glaucoma
- Congenital Glaucoma

10.1 INTRODUCTION

Glaucoma is a condition in which damage to the optic nerve occurs gradually. It is developed due to high ocular pressure. The function of the optic nerve is to transmit images of objects to the brain. If untreated, glaucoma can cause permanent optic nerve damage and vision loss. Glaucoma cannot be diagnosed easily as it may don't show any pain or symptoms of high eye pressure. Hence, it is recommended that the diagnosis of glaucoma is possible before losing the eyesight permanently.

According to the report of the World Health Organization, among the 2.2 billion people with impaired vision worldwide, it is conservatively estimated that at least 1 billion patients with moderate or severe far vision impairment or blindness could have been prevented or could still be cured, and 6.9 million people suffer from glaucoma among patients with moderate or severe far vision impairment or blindness.

10.1.1 The Definition of Glaucoma

Glaucoma is a group of diseases characterized by optic nerve *atrophy* and depression, visual field defect, and visual loss. *Pathological* elevated *intraocular* pressure and insufficient blood and nutrition supply to the optic nerve are the primary risk factors. Glaucoma is one of the three leading causes of blindness in human blindness. And the most important thing is the loss of vision caused by glaucoma is *irreversible*. The incidence rate is 1% in the general population and 2% in 45 years old.

10.1.2 Intraocular Pressure and Glaucoma
10.1.2.1 Anatomy and physiology

Key *anatomical* areas are the optic nerve, ciliary body, anterior chamber, and anterior chamber angle.

The *pathophysiology* of glaucoma revolves around aqueous humor dynamics. The main ocular structures related to it are the ciliary body, anterior chamber angle, and *aqueous outflow system*. The ciliary body is the area of aqueous production. The angle of the anterior chamber plays an important role in the process of aqueous *drainage*. It is formed by the root of the iris, the anterior-most part of the ciliary body, the *scleral spur*, *trabecular meshwork*, and Schwalbe's line. The angle width varies in different individuals and plays a vital role in the pathomechanism of different types of glaucoma. The angle structures can be visualized by gonioscopic examination (*Figure 10-1*).

10.1.2.2 Aqueous outflow system

It includes the trabecular meshwork, Schlemm's canal, collector channels, aqueous veins, and episcleral veins. Aqueous humor is derived from plasma within the capillary network of ciliary processes. The normal aqueous production rate is 2.3 μl/min. The trabecular meshwork is the main outlet for aqueous from the anterior chamber. Aqueous passes across the trabecular meshwork into the scheme's canal and is drained by collector channels. Approximately 90% of the total aqueous is drained out via this route. The *uveoscleral* outflow is responsible for about 7% of the total aqueous outflow. Aqueous passes across the ciliary body into the suprachoroidal space and is drained by the venous circulation in the ciliary body, choroid, and sclera. A little of aqueous is absorbed by the surface of the iris.

10.1.2.3 Intraocular pressure

The major risk factor for most glaucomas and the focus of treatment is increased intraocular pressure. Intraocular pressure is a function of the production of liquid aqueous humor by the ciliary processes of the eye and its drainage through the trabecular meshwork. Aqueous humor flows from the ciliary processes into the posterior chamber, bounded posteriorly by the lens and the zonules of Zinn and anteriorly by the iris. It then flows through the pupil of the iris into the anterior chamber, bounded posteriorly by the iris and anteriorly by the cornea. From here the trabecular meshwork drains aqueous humor via Schlemm's canal into scleral plexuses and general blood circulation.

Intraocular pressure is measured with a tonometer as part of a comprehensive eye examination. Measured values of intraocular pressure are influenced by corneal thickness and rigidity. As a result, some forms of refractive surgery (such as photorefractive keratectomy) can cause traditional intraocular pressure measurements to appear normal when the pressure may be abnormally high. Intraocular pressure (IOP) refers to the pressure exerted by intraocular fluids on the coats of the eyeball. The normal IOP varies between 10 and 21 mmHg (mean 16 ± 2.5 mmHg). The normal level of IOP is essentially maintained by a dynamic equilibrium between the inflow and outflow of the aqueous humor.

10.2 CLASSIFICATION OF GLAUCOMA

Glaucoma is clinically divided into three categories: primary, secondary, and *congenital* glaucoma. According to different pathogenesis, primary glaucoma is divided into *primary open-angle glaucoma (POAG)* and *primary angle closure glaucoma(PACG)*. Secondary glaucoma is not a disease caused by itself, but a group of diseases related to elevated intraocular pressure and some primary eye diseases or systemic diseases.

Clinico-etiologically glaucoma may be classified as follows:

1) Primary glaucoma

① Primary open-angle glaucoma (POAG).

② Primary angle closure glaucoma (PACG).

2) Secondary glaucoma

3) Congenital glaucoma

① Primary congenital glaucoma (without associated anomalies).

② Developmental glaucoma (with associated anomalies).

10.2.1 Primary Glaucoma
10.2.1.1 Signs and symptoms

There are two main types of primary glaucoma: primary open-angle glaucoma and primary-angle closure glaucoma.

POAG accounts for 90% of glaucoma cases in North America. It is painless and does not have acute attacks. The only signs are gradually progressive visual field loss, and optic nerve changes (increased cup-to-disc ratio on *fundoscopic examination*).

PACG accounts for less than 10% of glaucoma cases in North America, but as many as half of glaucoma cases in other nations (particularly Asian countries). About 10% of patients with closed angles present with acute angle-closure crises characterized by sudden ocular pain, seeing halos around lights, red eye, very high intraocular pressure (>30 mmHg), *nausea* and vomiting, sudden decreased vision, and a fixed, mid-dilated pupil. Acute angle closure is an ocular emergency.

10.2.1.2 Pathophysiology

In open-angle glaucoma, there is reduced flow through the trabecular meshwork; in angle-closure glaucoma, the *iridocorneal* angle is completely closed because of forward displacement of the final roll and root of the iris against the cornea resulting in the inability of the aqueous fluid to flow from the posterior to the anterior chamber and then out of the trabecular network.

The inconsistent relationship of glaucomatous optic neuropathy with ocular *hypertension* has provoked hypotheses and studies on anatomic structure, eye development, nerve compression trauma, optic nerve blood flow, excitatory *neurotransmitter*, trophic factor, retinal *ganglion* cell/axon degeneration, glial support cell, immune, aging mechanisms of neuron loss, and severing of the nerve fibers at the scleral edge, which results in characteristic optic disc appearance and specific visual field defects.

10.2.1.3 Etiological factors

Factors involved in the etiology of retinal ganglion cell death and thus in the etiology of glaucomatous optic neuropathy can be grouped as below.

1) Primary insults

① Elevated intraocular pressure: Elevated intraocular pressure leads to mechanical stretching of the sieve plate, which leads to *axonal* deformation and ischemia by changing capillary blood flow. Therefore, the neurotrophic factor (growth factor) cannot reach enough required for the survival of the retinal ganglion cell body.

② Pressure-independent factors: In glaucoma optic neuropathy in patients with normal intraocular pressure glaucoma, the factors affecting the vascular perfusion of the optic nerve head are involved without increasing intraocular pressure.

2) Secondary insults

Neuronal degeneration is driven by toxic factors, such as glutamate (excitatory toxin), oxygen-free radical, or nitric oxide, which is released when *retinal ganglion cells (RGCs)* die due to primary injury. In this way, even after the primary injury is controlled, the secondary injury will lead to sustained injury-mediated *apoptosis*.

10.2.1.4 Diagnosis

Screening for glaucoma is usually performed as part of a standard eye examination performed by ophthalmologists, orthoptists, and optometrists. Testing for glaucoma should include measurements of the intraocular pressure via tonometry, changes in size or shape of the eye, anterior chamber angle examination or *gonioscopy*, and examination of the optic nerve to look for any visible damage to it, or change in the *cup-to-disc ratio* and also rim appearance and vascular change. A formal visual field test should be performed. The *retinal nerve fiber layer* can be assessed with imaging techniques such as *optical coherence tomography (OCT)*, scanning laser polarimetry, and/or scanning laser ophthalmoscopy, also known as Heidelberg retina tomography (HRT).

Owing to the sensitivity of all methods of tonometry to corneal thickness, methods such as Goldmann tonometry should be augmented with pachymetry to measure central corneal thickness (CCT). A thicker-than-average cornea can result in a pressure reading higher than the "true" pressure, whereas a thinner-than-average cornea can produce a pressure reading lower than the "true" pressure.

Because pressure measurement error can be caused by more than just CCT (i.e. corneal hydration, elastic properties, etc.), it is impossible to "adjust" pressure measurements based only on CCT measurements. The Frequency Doubling Illusion can also be used to detect glaucoma with the use of a frequency doubling technology (FDT) perimeter.

Examination for glaucoma could also be assessed with more attention given to sex, race, history of drug use, refraction, inheritance, and family history.

10.2.1.5 Management

The modern goals of glaucoma management are to avoid glaucomatous damage and nerve damage and preserve the visual field and total quality of life for patients with minimal side effects. This requires appropriate diagnostic techniques follow-up examinations and judicious selection of treatments for the individual patient. Although intraocular pressure is only one of the major risk factors for glaucoma, lowering it via various pharmaceuticals and/ or surgical techniques is currently the mainstay of glaucoma treatment.

Vascular flow and *neurodegenerative* theories of glaucomatous optic neuropathy have prompted studies on various neuroprotective therapeutic strategies, including nutritional compounds, some of which may be regarded by clinicians as safe for use now, while others are on trial. The treatments are as follows.

1) Medication

There are three main ways to reduce intraocular pressure: increasing aqueous humor outflow, inhibiting aqueous humor generation, and reducing intraocular contents.

Intraocular pressure can be lowered with medication, usually eye drops. Several different classes of medications are used to treat glaucoma, with several different medications in each class.

Each of these medicines may have local and systemic side effects. Adherence to medication protocol can be confusing and expensive; if side effects occur, the patient must be willing either to tolerate these or to communicate with the treating physician to improve the drug regimen. Initially, glaucoma drops may reasonably be started in either one or both eyes.

Poor compliance with medications and follow-up visits is a major reason for vision loss in glaucoma patients. A 2003 study of patients in an HMO found that half failed to fill their prescriptions the first time, and one-fourth failed to refill their prescriptions a second time. Patient education and communication must be ongoing to sustain successful treatment plans for this lifelong disease with no early symptoms.

The possible neuroprotective effects of various topical and systemic medications are also being investigated.

2) *Trabeculectomy*

The most common conventional surgery performed for glaucoma is the trabeculectomy. Here, a partial thickness flap is made in the scleral wall of the eye, and a window opening is made under the flap to remove a portion of the trabecular meshwork. The scleral flap is then *sutured* loosely back in place to allow fluid to flow out of the eye through this opening, resulting in lowered intraocular pressure and the formation of a bleb or fluid bubble on the surface of the eye. Scarring can occur around or over the flap opening, causing it to become less effective or lose effectiveness altogether. Traditionally, chemotherapeutic adjuncts, such as *mitomycin* C or 5-fluorouracil, are applied with soaked sponges on the wound bed to prevent filtering blebs from scarring by inhibiting *fibroblast* proliferation. Contemporary alternatives include the sole or combinative implementation of non-chemotherapeutic adjuncts, such as collagen matrix implants or other biodegradable spacers, to prevent super scarring by randomization and modulation of fibroblast proliferation in addition to the mechanical prevention of wound contraction and adhesion.

3) Glaucoma drainage implants

Several different glaucoma drainage implants include the original Molteno implant (1966), the Baerveldt tube shunt, or the valved implants, such as the Ahmed glaucoma valve implant or the ExPress Mini Shunt and the later generation pressure ridge Molteno implants. These are indicated for glaucoma patients not responding to maximal medical therapy, with previous failed guarded filtering surgery (trabeculectomy). The flow tube is inserted into the anterior chamber of the eye, and the plate is implanted underneath the conjunctiva to allow the flow of aqueous fluid out of the eye into a chamber called a bleb.

The first-generation Molteno and other nonvalved implants sometimes require the ligation of the tube until the bleb formed is mildly fibrosed and watertight. This is done to reduce postoperative hypotony—sudden drops in postoperative intraocular pressure.

Valved implants, such as the Ahmed glaucoma valve, attempt to control postoperative hypotony by using a mechanical valve.

The ongoing scarring over the conjunctival dissipation segment of the shunt may become too thick for the aqueous humor to filter through. This may require preventive measures using antifibrotic medications, such as 5-fluorouracil or mitomycin-C (during the procedure), or other non-antifibrotic medication methods, such as collagen matrix implant, biodegradable spacer, or additional surgery. For glaucomatous painful blind eye and some cases of glaucoma, *cyclocryotherapy* for ciliary body ablation could be performed.

10.2.2 Secondary Glaucoma

Secondary glaucoma is a group of glaucoma with elevated intraocular pressure due to certain eye diseases or systemic diseases that disrupt aqueous humor circulation. Secondary glaucomas are named as follows:

- Lens-induced (phacogenic) glaucomas.
- *Inflammatory glaucoma* (glaucoma due to intraocular *inflammation*).
- *Pigmentary glaucoma.*
- *Neovascular glaucoma.*
- Glaucomas associated with irido-corneal *endothelial* syndromes.
- *Pseudoexfoliative glaucoma.*

- Glaucomas associated with intraocular *haemorrhage*.
- *Steroid-induced glaucoma.*
- *Traumatic glaucoma.*
- *Glaucoma-in-aphakia.*
- Glaucoma associated with intraocular tumours.

10.2.2.1 Lens-induced (phacogenic) glaucoma

1) Pathogenesis

① Phacomorphic glaucoma: The swollen lens pushes the iris forward and obliterates the angle resulting in secondary acute angle closure-glaucoma. Hence, the increased iridocorneal contact also causes potential pupillary block and iris bombe formation.

② Phacolytic glaucoma (Lens protein glaucoma) : This is a type of secondary open-angle glaucoma, in which trabecular meshwork is blocked by the proteins of the crystalline lens. Leakage of the lens proteins occurs through an intact capsule in the premature cataractous lens.

③ Lens particle glaucoma: This is a type of secondary open-angle glaucoma, in which trabecular meshwork is blocked by the lens particles floating in the aqueous humor.

2) Management

Medical therapy to lower IOP, irrigation-aspiration of the lens particles from the anterior chamber, or cataract extraction, which depends on the specific case.

10.2.2.2 Glaucomas due to uveitis

1) Pathogenesis

Iridocyclitis can lead to severe glaucoma, which is common in chronic cases. Inflammation leads to increased secretion of aqueous humor. During the inflammatory period, there is increased protein and cytokines in aqueous humor, leading to trabecular meshwork obstruction, or inflammation leads to secondary angle-closure with pupil block following iris bombe formation, or posterior synechia leads to pupil block, leading to increased intraocular pressure. The IOP can be raised by varied mechanisms in inflammations of the uveal tissue. Even in other ocular inflammations such as *keratitis* and *scleritis*, the rise in IOP is usually due to secondary involvement of the anterior uveal tract.

2) Management

It includes prophylaxis and curative treatment. Control eye inflammation and reduce intraocular pressure. Use mydriatic drops, *corticosteroids*, and eye drops for IOP lowering. Surgical or laser iridotomy may be useful in pupil block without angle closure. Filtration surgery may be performed in the presence of angle closure and IOP not in control.

10.2.2.3 Steroid-induced glaucoma

1) Pathogenesis

It is a type of secondary open-angle glaucoma that develops following long-term topical, and sometimes systemic *steroid* therapy. It leads to the collection of debris in the trabecular meshwork and decreases the aqueous outflow, or maybe the narrowing of trabecular spaces and a decrease in aqueous outflow, or leading to a decrease in aqueous outflow facility and an increase in IOP. In some cases, the IOP can be recovered after drug withdrawal, but in some cases, the IOP does not return to normal but increases after drug withdrawal.

2) Management

It can be prevented by the judicious use of steroids. Steroid drug users should use drugs under the guidance of doctors and closely monitor the changes in intraocular pressure. Those who are prone to induce high intraocular pressure reactions should be more careful to use corticosteroids. The principle of treatment is the same as that of primary open-angle glaucoma。

10.2.2.4 Neovascular glaucoma (NVG)

1) Pathogenesis

It is due to the formation of a neovascular membrane involving the angle of the anterior chamber. Based on primary ophthalmopathy, neovascularization appears in the iris. In the early stage of the disease, the outflow channel of aqueous humor is blocked by the neovascular membrane. In the late stage, the neovascular membrane shrinks and pulls, causing the closure of the angle and the increase of intraocular pressure with a lot of pain.

2) Management

① Injection of anti-VEGF, and panretinal photocoagulation may be carried out to prevent further neovascularization.

② Medical therapy and conventional filtration surgery are usually not effective in controlling the IOP. Artificial filtration shunt may control the IOP. Patients who cannot be solved finally can use eyeball enucleation.

10.2.2.5 Traumatic glaucoma

1) Pathogenesis

Blunt injuries and penetrating trauma of the eyeball can induce secondary glaucoma, and the most common is blunt injuries. When it comes to intraocular hemorrhage, especially vitreous hemorrhage, sometimes these can induce hemorrhagic glaucoma and ghost-cell glaucoma. Because of intraocular hemorrhage, red blood cells accumulate on the trabecular meshwork, blood clots block the pupil, or inflammatory edema on trabecular meshwork can cause aqueous humor drainage blocked. After several months or years of eyeball blunt injuries, angle-reduction glaucoma may also occur, which is similar to POAG and the treatment principle is the same with POAG.

2) Management

Medical therapy with topical timolol and oral *acetazolamide*, treatment of associated causative mechanism, and surgical intervention according to the situation. If the conservative treatment is not effective, the patient can be treated with anterior chamber inversion or *vitrectomy*.

10.2.3 Congenital Glaucoma

Congenital glaucoma is a disease that leads to abnormally high intraocular pressure due to abnormal development of anterior chamber angle obstructing the aqueous humor drainage during *embryonic* and developmental stages. This is a rare condition seen in newborn babies and children. Congenital glaucoma causes complete blindness, if it is not diagnosed and left untreated. Sometimes glaucoma may occur several years after birth. It can be divided into 2 types: primary infantile/juvenile glaucoma; and developmental glaucoma with associated ocular anomalies.

10.2.3.1 Primary infantile/juvenile glaucoma

1) Signs and Symptoms

Photophobia, *blepharospasm*, and *lacrimation* are essential features. Corneal signs include *edema*, enlargement, and Descemet's breaks called Haab's striae. And the *anterior chamber depth* changes deeper with time. Elevated intraocular pressure, and abnormal anterior chamber angle, which you can use ophthalmoscopy to evaluate the optic disc.

2) Pathophysiology

The attachment point of the iris root moves forward, and too much iris root covers the surface of the trabeculum, resulting in the lack of *permeability* of trabecular meshwork that is responsible for blocking aqueous outflow resulting in raised IOP.

3) Prevalence and genetic pattern

About 10% of the cases show an autosomal recessive inheritance, with incomplete penetrance, or polygenic inheritance. 65% of the patients are boys. The disease is bilateral in 75% of cases, but the involvement may be *asymmetric* and *asynchronous*.

4) Diagnosis

① Tonometry: Measurement of intraocular pressure by using applanation tonometers, such as Perkins and Tono-pen.

② Cornea: *Cloudy cornea*, *Haab's striae* presence and corneal diameter lager than 11 mm at birth.

③ Gonioscopy: Maldevelopment of trabeculum and anterior chamber angle is open.

④ Fundus: C/D ratio(cup/disk ratio) is lager than 0.3 and atrophy.

5) Management

Treatment of primary infantile/juvenile glaucoma is goniotomy or trabeculotomy. However, if it occurs in juveniles, patients can be treated with drugs at first.

10.2.3.2 Developmental glaucoma with associated ocular anomalies

It is usually associated with systemic abnormalities and ocular anomalies, such as Marfan's syndrome, Sturge-Weber syndrome, and Axenfeld-Rieger syndrome. These diseases mainly depend on surgical treatment, and in the meantime manage other congenital abnormalities, often with a poor prognosis.

Chapter 11
Diseases of the Uveal Tract

INTRODUCTION
UVEITIS
  ▶ Anterior Uveitis
  ▶ Intermediate Uveitis
  ▶ Posterior Uveitis
  ▶ Panuveitis
  ▶ Several Noninfectious Uveitis
CONGENITAL ABNORMALITIES OF THE UVEAL TRACT
  ▶ Aniridia
  ▶ Coloboma of the Iris
  ▶ Persistent Pupillary Membrane
  ▶ Coloboma of the Choroid

11.1 INTRODUCTION

The uveal tract is a part of the eye that consists of three structures: the iris, ciliary body, and choroid. It plays a crucial role in maintaining the health and function of the eye. This chapter focuses on various diseases that affect the uveal tract and their classifications.

Uveitis is a potentially serious condition that can lead to vision loss if not diagnosed and treated promptly. Uveitis can be classified based on various factors, including the location of inflammation within the uveal tract and the duration of the disease.

11.2 UVEITIS

Uveitis used to refer to inflammation of the uvea itself, but currently internationally, inflammation that occurs in the uvea, retinal blood vessels, and vitreous body is commonly referred to as uveitis as well. Some people also classify inflammation of the optic papilla as uveitis. Uveitis often occurs in young adults and is prone to systemic autoimmune diseases. It often recurs and is difficult to treat, leading to serious complications. It is a common and important type of blinding eye disease.

Although there are currently multiple classification methods for uveitis, there is no satisfactory classification method. The commonly used classification methods include the following:

① Etiological classification can be divided into two categories: infectious and non-infectious according to the cause of the disease. The former include infections caused by *bacteria*, *fungi*, *spirochetes*, viral parasites, etc., while the latter includes types such as idiopathic, *traumatic*, autoimmune, *rheumatic* diseases accompanied by uveitis, *camouflage syndrome*, etc.

②Clinical and pathological classification: According to the clinical and histological changes of inflammation, it can be divided into *granulomatous* and non-granulomatous uveitis. Previously, it was believed that granulomatous inflammation was mainly related to *pathogen* infection, rather than granulomatous inflammation and allergies. In fact, both infectious and non-infectious factors can cause two types of inflammation, and some types of uveitis can manifest as either granulomatous or non-granulomatous inflammation at different stages and individuals of the disease.

③Anatomical position classification: This classification method was developed by the International Group on Uveitis (1979) and recognized by the International Society of Ophthalmology. Recently, the International Working Group on Uveitis Nomenclature has made modifications and improvements to this classification method. According to anatomical location, uveitis can be divided into *anterior uveitis*, *intermediate uveitis*, *posterior uveitis*, and total uveitis. A disease course of less than 3 months is acute inflammation, and a disease course of more than 3 months is chronic inflammation.

11.2.1 Anterior Uveitis

Anterior uveitis includes three types: *iritis*, *iridocyclitis*, and anterior ciliary inflammation. It is the most common type of uveitis, accounting for about 50% of the total number of uveitis in China.

From the perspective of etiology and course, anterior uveitis can be roughly divided into three categories: *acute anterior uveitis*, which is often HLA-B27 positive and can be combined with *ankylosing spondylitis*, *psoriatic arthritis*, *reactive arthritis*, and inflammatory intestinal diseases; chronic anterior uveitis such as Fuchs syndrome and white uveitis in children; both acute and chronic inflammation can occur, such as *juvenile idiopathic arthritis*, *tuberculosis* and *syphilis*, which can cause such inflammation.

11.2.1.1 Clinical manifestations of anterior uveitis

1) Symptoms

Acute inflammation can cause eye pain, photophobia, tearing, and blurred vision. When there is a large amount of fibrin exudation reactive macular edema or optic disc edema in the anterior chamber, visual acuity may decrease or significantly decrease. In chronic inflammation, the symptoms may not be obvious, but it is prone to concurrent cataracts or secondary glaucoma, which can lead to severe visual impairment.

2) Physical signs

① Ciliary congestion or mixed congestion: Ciliary congestion refers to the congestion of superficial scleral blood vessels located around the corneal margin, and is a common sign of acute anterior uveitis. But *keratitis* and acute angle-closure glaucoma can also cause such congestion, and attention should be paid to differentiation.

② *Keratic precipitates (KP)* are inflammatory cells or pigments that deposit on the posterior surface of the cornea, known as KP. Its formation requires the simultaneous presence of corneal endothelial damage and inflammatory cells or pigments. According to the shape of KP, it can be divided into three types, namely dust-like, medium-sized, and mutton fat-like. The first two are mainly composed of *neutrophils*, *lymphocytes*, and *plasma cells*, while the latter are mainly composed of monocyte *macrophages* and epithelioid cells. Dust-like KP is mainly seen in non-granulomatous anterior uveitis, and can also be seen at a certain stage of granulomatous uveitis; Moderate size KP is mainly seen in anterior uveitis associated with Fuchs syndrome and viral keratitis; Mutton fat like KP is mainly seen in granulomatous uveitis.

KP has three types of distribution:

- The triangular distribution below, which is the most common form of distribution;
- The distribution of corneal foramen is mainly seen in Fuchs syndrome, glaucoma, ciliary body inflammation syndrome, and anterior uveitis accompanied by toxic keratitis;
- Diffuse distribution behind the cornea, mainly seen in anterior uveitis accompanied by Fuchs syndrome and viral keratitis.

③ *Anterior chamber flare*: It is caused by the disruption of the blood-aqueous barrier function and the entry of proteins into the aqueous humor. During slit lamp examination, it appears as a white beam in the anterior chamber. Active anterior uveitis often causes anterior chamber flare. After the anterior uveitis subsides, the damage to the blood-queous barrier function may take some time to recover, so there may still be anterior chamber flare. Acute angle-closure glaucoma and ocular contusion can also cause damage to the blood-aqueous barrier function, leading to anterior chamber flare. Therefore, anterior chamber flare does not necessarily represent active inflammation, nor is it an indication of local use of *glucocorticoids*.

④ Anterior chamber cells: Under pathological conditions, inflammatory cells, red blood cells, tumor cells, or pigment cells can appear in the aqueous humor. During uveitis, the main cells are inflammatory cells. On slit lamp examination, uniform gray-white dust-like particles can be seen, with upward movement near the iris and downward movement near the corneal surface. Inflammatory cells are reliable indicators of anterior segment inflammation. When a large number of inflammatory cells deposit in the lower chamber corner of the aqueous humor, they can be seen at the liquid level, which is called *hypopyon*. When inflammation is severe, a large amount of fibrous exudation can occur, causing the aqueous humor to be in a relatively solidified state.

⑤ Iris changes: The iris can undergo various changes, and the fibrous exudation and *proliferation* on the anterior surface of the iris and lens can cause them to adhere together, known as the posterior *synechia* of the iris. If there is extensive posterior synechia of the iris, the aqueous humor cannot flow from the posterior chamber to the anterior chamber, resulting in an increase in posterior chamber pressure. The iris is pushed forward and becomes swollen, known as iris bombe; The *adhesion* between the iris and the posterior surface of the cornea is called anterior synechia of the iris. If this adhesion occurs at the angle of the atrium, it is called *goniosynechia*. Inflammatory damage can cause changes such as *depigmentation*, atrophy, and discoloration of the iris. Inflammation can cause three types of *nodules*: Koeppe nodules, which occur at the pupil margin and can be seen in non-granulomatous and granulomatous inflammations; Busacca nodules are white or grayish-white *translucent* nodules that occur within the iris *parenchyma*, mainly seen in granulomatous inflammation; Iris granuloma is a pink opaque nodule that occurs in the iris parenchyma, mainly seen in anterior uveitis caused by sarcoidosis.

⑥ Pupil changes: During inflammation, due to the spasm of ciliary muscle and the continuous contraction of the *sphincter* of the pupil, the pupil may shrink. The posterior synechia of the iris cannot be opened, and after *mydriasis*, there are often many shapes of pupil appearance, such as plum blossom, pear or irregular, and if the iris has 360 ° synechia, it is called pupillary *atresia*; If the fibrous *membrane* covers the entire pupil area, it is called *occlusion of pupil*.

⑦ Lens changes: During anterior uveitis, pigments can deposit on the anterior surface of the lens. When the fresh posterior adhesion of the iris is removed, circular pigments can be left on the anterior surface of the lens.

⑧ Changes in the vitreous body and posterior segment of the eye: Inflammatory cells can appear in the anterior vitreous body during iris ciliary inflammation and anterior ciliary inflammation, while in patients with simple iritis, there are generally no inflammatory cells in the anterior vitreous body. Anterior uveitis generally does not have vitreous opacity, but occasionally reactive macular cystoid edema or optic disc edema may occur.

11.2.1.2 Complications of anterior uveitis

① Recurrent or chronic inflammation of concurrent cataracts can cause changes in aqueous humor, affect lens metabolism, and cause cataracts, often manifested as posterior *subcapsular* opacities. In addition, during anterior uveitis, long-term use of glucocorticoid eye drops can also cause posterior subcapsular opacity of the lens.

② When secondary glaucoma is caused by anterior uveitis, elevated intraocular pressure or secondary glaucoma can be caused by the following factors: a. inflammatory cells, fibrous exudation, and tissue debris blocking the trabecular meshwork; b. inflammation of the anterior adhesion or trabecular meshwork around the iris, which hinders the drainage of aqueous humor; c. pupil atresia and pupillary membrane closure blocking the entry of aqueous humor from the posterior chamber into the anterior chamber.

③ Low intraocular pressure and recurrent or chronic inflammation of eyeball atrophy can lead to detachment or atrophy of the ciliary body, decreased secretion of aqueous humor, and a decrease in intraocular pressure. In severe cases, it can lead to eyeball atrophy.

11.2.1.3 Acute anterior uveitis (AAU)

It presents with sudden-onset inflammation of the iris and anterior chamber. It is often associated with pain, redness, and sensitivity to light.

1) Clinical manifestations

Usually, there are symptoms such as sudden eye pain, redness, photophobia, and tearing. During the examination, ciliary congestion, dusty KP, obvious anterior chamber flare, and a large number of anterior chamber cells can be seen, which can be accompanied by changes such as fiber exudation, anterior chamber pus accumulation, pupil narrowing, and posterior iris adhesions.

2) Diagnosis

Based on the patient's clinical manifestations. Due to the fact that various systemic diseases can cause or accompany this type of uveitis, determining the etiology and accompanying diseases is of great value in guiding treatment and predicting prognosis. Therefore, for acute anterior uveitis, a detailed medical history should be inquired, especially whether there are systemic diseases such as low back pain, joint redness and swelling, *urethritis*, *digestive tract* abnormalities, *respiratory system* abnormalities, psoriasis, skin lesions, etc., to determine whether there is ankylosing spondylitis, reactive arthritis, inflammatory bowel disease, psoriatic arthritis, tuberculosis, and syphilis. Laboratory tests include blood routine, erythrocyte sedimentation rate, HLA-B27 antigen typing, etc. For those suspected to be caused by pathogen infection, corresponding etiological tests should be conducted.

3) Differential diagnosis

① Acute conjunctivitis presents as an acute onset, with foreign body sensation, burning sensation, and excessive secretion. Examination shows swelling of the eyes and face, and conjunctival congestion, which are significantly different from the symptoms of photophobia, tearing, blurred vision, ciliary congestion, and anterior chamber inflammation in acute anterior uveitis.

② Acute angle-closure glaucoma presents with acute onset, sudden decrease in vision, headache, nausea, vomiting, corneal epithelial edema, corneal haze, shallow anterior chamber, anterior chamber flare, etc., but without anterior chamber inflammatory cells. The pupils are oval-shaped and dilated, with increased intraocular pressure. It is easy to distinguish between acute anterior uveitis and acute anterior uveitis with transparent cornea, a large amount of KP, normal anterior chamber depth, abundant inflammatory cells in aqueous humor, reduced pupils, and normal or low intraocular pressure.

③ Differentiate some types of uveitis from total uveitis, which can cause anterior uveitis, such as Behcet's disease with uveitis Vogt Kobayashi Harada's disease at a certain stage, which can all manifest as anterior uveitis. However, these two types of uveitis are often accompanied by extraocular manifestations, so attention should be paid to differentiation in diagnosis.

4) Treatment

The treatment principle is to immediately dilate the pupils to prevent and retract fresh iris adhesion and quickly anti-inflammatory to prevent eye tissue from being damaged and complications. Due to the vast majority of anterior uveitis being caused by non-infectious factors, antibiotic treatment is generally not required. For highly suspected or confirmed cases of pathogen infection, corresponding anti-infective treatment should be given. For uveitis caused by non-infectious factors, as local medication can reach an effective concentration in the anterior segment, systemic medication is generally not necessary. However, when anterior chamber inflammation is severe, glucocorticoid injection around the eye or short-term systemic treatment can be given.

① The frequency of glucocorticoid eye drops should be determined according to the severity of inflammation. Patients with papilledema and macular edema can be treated with glucocorticoid orally for a short time.

② *Cycloplegic* agent. Usually post atropine eye ointment or eye drops are used. For patients with severe inflammation, 1% atropine eye drops can be used first, and then post-atropine or short-acting cycloplegic eye drops can be used after the inflammation is curbed.

③ NSAIDs eye drops.

④ Treat concomitant systemic diseases.

⑤ Refractory inflammation may be treated with other *immunosuppressant*.

⑥ Etiological treatment.

⑦ Treatment of complications, such as anti-glaucoma surgery, cataract extraction, and intraocular lens implantation

11.2.1.4 Chronic anterior uveitis

This form of uveitis has a more prolonged course, with less severe symptoms compared to acute anterior uveitis.

1) Clinical manifestations

Patients often have no or mild ciliary congestion, and KP can be dust-like, medium-sized, or mutton fat-like. Koeppe nodules and/or Busacca nodules, iris depigmentation, atrophy, and posterior adhesions may appear, and complications such as cataracts and secondary glaucoma may occur.

2) Diagnosis

It is generally easy to diagnose based on clinical manifestations, but attention should be paid to combined systemic diseases, especially those that occur under the age of 16. A detailed history of arthritis, rash, and other diseases should be inquired about, and anti-nuclear antibody tests should be conducted to determine whether juvenile idiopathic arthritis is combined.

3) Treatment

Corticosteroids and cycloplegics are commonly used local treatment drugs (see treatment for acute anterior uveitis), but the frequency of eye drops should depend on the severity of the inflammation. For patients with concomitant systemic diseases such as juvenile idiopathic arthritis, inflammatory bowel disease, and Vogt Kobayashi Harada disease, in addition to local medication, systemic use of corticosteroids and/or other immunosuppressants is also necessary.

11.2.2 Intermediate Uveitis

Intermediate uveitis is a group of inflammatory and proliferative diseases that involve the flat part of the ciliary body, the basal part of the vitreous body, the surrounding retina, and the choroid. In previous literature, this disease has multiple names, such as posterior ciliary body inflammation, chronic posterior ciliary body inflammation, ciliary planitis, or peripheral uveitis. The International Uveitis Research Group has uniformly named this type of disease intermediate uveitis. It is more common in people under the age of 40, with a similar incidence rate between men and women. It often affects both eyes and can occur simultaneously or sequentially. Usually manifested as a chronic inflammatory process.

11.2.2.1 Clinical manifestation

① The onset of symptoms is hidden, and the exact onset time cannot be determined. Mild cases may have no symptoms or only *floaters*, while severe cases may have blurred vision or temporary myopia; When the macula is affected or cataracts appear, there may be a significant decrease in vision, and a few patients may experience symptoms such as redness and eye pain.

② The most common changes are vitreous snowball opacity, snowbank-like changes in the flattened part of the ciliary body, peripheral retinal vein inflammation, and inflammatory lesions. At the same time, anterior segment involvement and posterior pole retinal changes can also occur.

Changes in the anterior segment: There may be mutton fat or dusty KP, mild anterior chamber flare, a small to moderate amount of anterior chamber cells, posterior iris adhesions, anterior adhesions, and goniosynechia. In children, symptoms of acute anterior uveitis such as ciliary congestion and a large number of inflammatory cells in the aqueous humor can appear.

Retinal and choroidal damage: Retinitis in the lower peripheral area, retinal *vasculitis*, and peripheral retinal choroiditis can occur.

11.2.2.2 Complications

Cystic edema of the macula is the most common, and changes such as macular membrane and macular hole can also occur. Maculopathy; Complicated cataracts are common, mainly manifested as posterior subcapsular opacities; Other retinal *neovascularization*, vitreous hemorrhage, *proliferative vitreoretinopathy*, optic disc edema, or optic nerve atrophy can also occur.

11.2.2.3 Diagnosis

Based on typical vitreous snowball opacity, snowbank-like changes, and peripheral retinal vasculitis below. However, in clinical practice, it is prone to misdiagnosis or missed diagnosis, so detailed examination should be conducted. Binocular indirect ophthalmoscope and peripheral fundus examination should be performed for the following situations: The occurrence of floaters and the tendency to worsen; Posterior subcapsular opacification due to other reasons that are difficult to explain; *Cystic macular edema* that cannot be explained by other reasons. FFA examination can detect changes such as retinal vasculitis, macular cystoid edema, and optic disc edema, which is helpful for diagnosis.

11.2.2.4 Treatment

① Those with visual acuity greater than 0.5 are usually followed up.

② Glucocorticoids can be given eye drops, posterior tenon subcapsular injection, or oral administration according to the situation.

③ Other immunosuppressants can be selected, such as chlorambucil, cyclophosphamide, etc.

④ If the drug treatment effect is not good, if there is a snowbank-like lesion in the flat part of the ciliary body, the condensation treatment of the flat part of the ciliary body is feasible.

⑤ Vitrectomy is feasible for those who fail to respond to the above treatment.

⑥ Retinal neovascularization can be treated by *laser photocoagulation*.

⑦ Patients with anterior chamber inflammation should be treated with cycloplegic agents and NSAIDs.

11.2.3 Posterior Uveitis

Posterior uveitis is a group of inflammatory diseases that involve the choroid, retina, retinal blood vessels, and vitreous body. Clinically, it includes choroiditis, retinitis, chorioretinitis, and retinal vasculitis.

11.2.3.1 Clinical manifestation

① Symptoms: Mainly depend on the type, affected area, and severity of inflammation. May have dark shadows or dark spots, flashes, or visual changes. Those with blurred appearance, blurred vision, or decreased vision, combined with systemic diseases, have corresponding systemic symptoms.

② The physical signs: Depend on the location and severity of inflammation. Common ones include inflammatory cells and *turbidity* in the vitreous body; *Focal chorioretinal infiltration lesions*, which may vary in size, and may form a cicatrization in the later stage; Diffuse choroiditis; Retinal vasculitis, including vascular sheath, vascular occlusion, and bleeding; Retinal edema or macular edema. In addition, there may also be changes such as exudative retinal detachment, proliferative vitreoretinopathy, retinal neovascularization, choroidal neovascularization, or vitreous hemorrhage. Generally, there is no change in the anterior segment, but occasionally there may be anterior chamber flare and a small amount of inflammatory cells in the aqueous humor.

11.2.3.2 Diagnosis

Based on typical clinical manifestations, a diagnosis can be made. FFA is of great help in identifying retinal and vasculitis, as well as choroidal pigment epithelial lesions, while ICGA is helpful in identifying choroidal and vascular lesions. B-mode ultrasound, OCT, CT, and MRI may all be helpful in determining the lesions caused by inflammation or in tracing the cause. Corresponding laboratory tests can be selected based on the patient's clinical manifestations.

11.2.3.3 Treatment

① If confirmed to be caused by infectious factors, corresponding anti-infective treatment should be given.

② Inflammation caused by immune factors is mainly treated with immunosuppressive agents.

③ Unilaterally affected individuals can be treated with glucocorticoid followed by tenon subcapsular injection.

④ For patients with bilateral or unilateral involvement, it is not advisable to undergo tenon subcapsular injection. They should take corticosteroids, phenylbutyrate nitrogen mustard, or cyclophosphamide. Due to the stubborn nature of some types of posterior uveitis, immunosuppressive agents should be used for a sufficient period of time. Combined use can often reduce the side effects of drugs and enhance their efficacy. During the treatment process, liver and kidney function, blood routine, blood sugar, etc. should be regularly checked to avoid serious drug toxicity and side effects.

⑤ For patients with retinal neovascularization or choroidal neovascularization, treatment such as invitation photocoagulation and anti-VEGF therapy may be considered.

11.2.4 Panuveitis

Generalized uveitis (or *panuveitis*) refers to inflammation that affects the entire uvea, often accompanied by inflammation of the retina and vitreous body. When inflammation caused by infectious factors mainly occurs in the vitreous or aqueous humor, it is called endophthalmitis.

11.2.4.1 Clinical manifestation

① There may be obvious redness, eye pain, photophobia, tears, floaters, flashes, blurred vision, or decreased vision, or there may be no obvious symptoms of iridocyclitis.

② With or without ciliary congestion, dust-like or mutton fat-like KP, anterior chamber flare, inflammatory cells in aqueous humor, hypopyon, iris nodules, posterior iris adhesions, etc.

③ Vitreous inflammatory cells, turbidity, and fibroproliferative membranes.

④ Retinitis, necrotic focus, or retinal choroid inflammatory focus.

⑤ Punctate or patchy, single or multiple foci of choroidal inflammation, with scar formation in the late stage.

⑥ Retinal vasculitis, perivasculitis, vascular occlusion, neovascularization, etc.

⑦ It can be accompanied by macular edema, papilledema, etc.

⑧ Systemic manifestations of comorbidities.

11.2.4.2 Diagnosis

① Clinical features of anterior and posterior uveitis.

② History or clinical manifestations of systemic diseases.

③ FFA showed retinitis, retinal vasculitis, choroiditis, retinal pigment epithelial lesions, hemorrhage, neovascularization, etc.

④ ICGA showed choroidal vasodilation, leakage, etc.

⑤ Perform corresponding laboratory tests to determine the etiology or type.

11.2.4.3 Treatment

① Etiological treatment.

② Glucocorticoid treatment should be given the appropriate dose according to the type of inflammation, and the appropriate treatment time should be selected through the appropriate way for standardized treatment.

③ For those with poor therapeutic effect of glucocorticoids or intractable inflammation, other immunosuppressants should be selected according to the patient's situation, and the side effects of drugs should be paid attention to during the treatment.

④ In case of complications, corresponding treatment should be carried out.

11.2.5 Several Noninfectious Uveitis

11.2.5.1 Ankylosing spondylitis

Ankylosing spondylitis is an idiopathic inflammatory disease whose etiology is not completely clear, mainly involving the axial bone joints. About 20%~25% of patients develop acute anterior uveitis.

1) Clinical manifestation

① More male patients than female patients.

② Multiple eyes are involved, but both eyes often have alternating attacks.

③ The vast majority are acute anterior uveitis.

④ The vast majority are non-granulomatous inflammation. Uveitis tends to recur.

⑤ Pain and stiffness in the waist, especially in the morning, will be relieved after exercise, and the spine will be stiff in the late stage.

2) Diagnosis

① Typical history of anterior uveitis and lumbosacral pain.

② X-ray examination showed sacroiliitis and spinal ankylosis changes.

③ HLA-B27 positive.

11.2.5.2 Vogt Koyanagi Harada syndrome

Vogt Koyanagi Harada (VKH) syndrome, also known as idiopathic Uvea encephalitis, is characterized by bilateral diffuse exudative uveitis, accompanied by systemic meningeal irritation, hearing impairment, vitiligo, hair whitening or shedding, and other diseases. The pathological manifestation is chronic diffuse granuloma uveitis. This disease is related to *autoimmune* and genetic factors, with a significant increase in HLA-BW54.

1) Clinical manifestation

① Precursory symptoms include headache, neck stiffness, *tinnitus*, hearing loss, scalp allergy, etc.

② At the beginning of the disease, bilateral diffuse choroiditis, neuro retinitis optica, retinal edema at the posterior pole, or even serous retinal detachment occur.

③ If the disease is not effectively controlled, the anterior uvea may be involved, such as dusty or mutton fat KP, anterior chamber flare, aqueous humor inflammatory cells, iris nodules, posterior synechia of the iris, or even pupillary atresia.

④ *Recurrent granuloma panuveitis*, sunset-like fundus, Dalen-Fuchs nodules.

⑤ Hair loss, hair whitening, vitiligo, hearing loss, tinnitus.

⑥ Complications such as secondary glaucoma and concurrent cataracts are prone to occur.

2) Diagnosis

Based on the medical history and clinical manifestations, combined with the overall condition, the diagnosis can be made. The presence of pigment epithelial damage and multiple punctate high *fluorescence* features during the acute inflammatory phase of fundus fluorescence imaging is of great help in diagnosis. Dalen-Fuchs nodules are typical features of Vogt Kobayashi Harada syndrome and *sympathetic ophthalmia*, and a diagnosis can be made by ruling out eye trauma and a history of internal eye surgery. When laboratory examination of cerebrospinal fluid reveals lymphocyte proliferation, it can assist in diagnosis.

11.2.5.3 Behcet disease

This disease is a chronic persistent disease that affects multiple organs of the body. The main pathological change is obliterative vasculitis. It is clinically characterized by uveitis, *aphthous* stomatitis, skin damage, and ulcers of the vulva. This disease mainly occurs in some countries along the Far East, Middle East, and Mediterranean coast, and is also common in China. At present, the cause is unknown. Patients with this disease often have a variety of autoantibodies, so it may be an autoimmune disease, or it may be caused by an autoimmune reaction induced by virus infection. This disease has a clear genetic background, with HLA-B5 exceeding the norm by times, and eye inflammation being significantly more correlated.

1) Clinical manifestation

① Ocular lesions: Non-granulomatous recurrent panuveitis. The patient has photophobia, tears, pain, vision loss, and other symptoms. Ocular examination reveals ciliary congestion, KP, aqueous humor opacification, hypopyon, posterior iris synechia, vitreous opacification, retinal choroidal exudation foci, vascular migration and hemorrhage, etc. Retinal vascular closure is more common in the later stage. The common complications are complicated cataracts, secondary glaucoma, proliferative retinopathy, and optic atrophy.

② Systemic lesions can be complicated by multiple recurrent oral ulcers, skin erythema nodosa, acne-like rash, etc. Nodules and shriveled rash (positive skin allergic reaction) appear at the place of *acupuncture*, which is the characteristic change of this disease. Others include joint swelling, *thrombophlebitis*, nervous system damage, peptic ulcer, genital ulcer, etc.

2) Diagnosis

The diagnosis is mainly based on the ocular characteristics and the manifestations of systemic complications. The International Uveitis Research Group recommends the following diagnostic criteria:

① Recurrent oral ulcer recurred at least 3 times within 1 year.

② The disease can be confirmed if two of the following four items occur: a. recurrent genital ulcer or scar; b. uveitis changes in the eye; c. erythema nodosum, pseudofolliculitis or purulent papule in the skin; d. positive skin allergic reaction test.

11.2.5.4 Fuchs heterochromic uveitis

Fuchs heterochromic uveitis is a chronic non-granulomatous uveitis characterized by iris depigmentation. 90% of patients have monocular involvement. The main manifestation is anterior uveitis, and the vitreous and peripheral retina can also be involved.

1) Clinical manifestation

① Decreased vision, or blurred vision.

② No symptoms and signs of acute iridocyclitis.

③ Medium-sized KP or star-shaped KP, with triangular distribution, pupil area distribution, or diffuse distribution behind the cornea.

④ Mild anterior chamber flare and a few inflammatory cells.

⑤ Iris depigmentation or atrophy.

⑥ Koeppe nodules often appear.

⑦ Posterior subcapsular opacification and elevated intraocular pressure.

⑧ Pre vitreous opacities and cells may appear.

⑨ Inflammatory lesions of the lower peripheral retina and choroid can be seen in a few patients.

2) Diagnosis

① No symptoms and signs of acute anterior uveitis.

② Mild non-granulomatous anterior uveitis.

③ Characteristic KP.

④ Iris depigmentation.

11.2.5.5 Sympathetic ophthalmia

Sympathetic ophthalmia refers to bilateral granulomatous uveitis that occurs after perforation of one eye or internal eye surgery. The injured eye is called the induced eye, and the other eye is called the sympathetic eye. It is mainly caused by the exposure of intraocular antigens and the stimulation of autoimmune response caused by trauma or surgery.

1) Clinical manifestations

It can occur within 5 days to 56 years after trauma or surgery, but most of it occurs within 2 weeks to 2 months. The disease is generally occult, mostly granulomatous inflammation. There may be sunset-like fundus and Dalen Fuchs nodules similar to Vogt Koyanagi Harada disease, as well as some extraocular lesions such as vitiligo, alopecia, hearing loss, or meningeal irritation.

2) Diagnosis

The history of ocular perforation or internal eye surgery is of great value in the diagnosis of this disease and is also an important basis for differentiating it from Vogt Koyanagi Harada disease. FFA examination showed early multifocal leakage and late dye accumulation, which may be accompanied by optic disc staining.

11.3 CONGENITAL ABNORMALITIES OF THE UVEAL TRACT

Congenital abnormalities of the uvea are often related to incomplete closure of *embryonic* fissures during the development of early embryonic eyes.

11.3.1 Aniridia

Aniridia is a rare congenital malformation of the eye, almost always involving both eyes. Often accompanied by abnormalities in the cornea, anterior chamber, crystalline retina, and optic nerve, it belongs to *autosomal* dominant inheritance. The iris is completely missing, and the equatorial edge of the lens, suspensory *ligament*, and ciliary process can be directly seen. There may be low vision caused by photophobia and various eye abnormalities, and many patients may become blind due to progressive corneal/lens opacity, or glaucoma. To reduce photophobia and discomfort, colored glasses or contact lenses can be worn.

11.3.2 Coloboma of the Iris

Coloboma of the iris are divided into two types: typical and simple defects. The typical coloboma of the iris is a complete coloboma of the iris located below, forming a pear-shaped pupil with the tip downward. The difference from the surgical excision is that the edge of the defect is covered by pigment epithelium, which is often accompanied by other congenital eye malformations, such as a ciliary body or choroidal defect. Simple coloboma of the iris refers to coloboma of the iris that does not merge with other uveal abnormalities, manifested as pupil edge notch, iris hole, iris peripheral defect, iris matrix, and pigment epithelial defect, etc. and does not affect vision.

11.3.3 Persistent Pupillary Membrane

A persistent pupillary membrane is a residue of incomplete absorption of the vascular membrane on the surface of the embryonic lens. There are two types: filamentous and membranous, with one end starting from the iris ring and the other end attached to the opposite iris ring, or attached to the anterior capsule of the lens. It usually does not affect vision and pupil activity and does not require treatment. For thicker pupillary membranes that affect vision, surgery or laser treatment is feasible.

11.3.4 Coloboma of the Choroid

Coloboma of the choroid are divided into two types: typical and *atypical*. Typical choroidal defects often occur in both eyes, located below the optic disc nose and also including the optic disc. The defect area is characterized by a lack of choroid, with a transparent white sclera visible through the thin retina. The edges are mostly neat and pigmented, often accompanied by microphthalmos, iris abnormalities, optic nerve abnormalities, lens absence, and abnormal development of the macula. Atypical defects are relatively rare, mostly monocular, and can be located in any part of the fundus, with macular area defects being the most common and central visual loss, similar to typical cases. There is no specific treatment. Surgery is feasible when complicated with retinal detachment.

Chapter 12
Lens Diseases

INTRODUCTION

CATARACT
- ▶ Etiology and Pathogenesis of Cataract
- ▶ Classification
- ▶ Clinical Manifestation
- ▶ Congenital and Developmental Cataract
- ▶ Acquired Cataract
- ▶ Posterior Capsular Opacification

MANAGEMENT OF CATARACT
- ▶ Surgical Indications and Surgical Contraindications
- ▶ Preoperative Examination
- ▶ Phacoemulsification
- ▶ Intraocular Lens Options
- ▶ Complications of Cataract Surgery and Management

DISLOCATED LENS (ECTOPIA LENTIS)
- ▶ Definition
- ▶ Etiology
- ▶ Lens Subluxation
- ▶ Lens Luxation

CONGENITAL ANOMALIES OF THE LENS
- ▶ Abnormal Lens Formation
- ▶ Abnormal Lens Morphology

12.1 INTRODUCTION

The lens is located between the iris, pupil, and vitreous body. It is shaped like a convex lens and completely transparent. The lens has strong refractive power and is an important part of the refractive interstitium. Diseases of the lens include *cataracts*, dislocation of the lens, congenital *malformations* of the lens, and aphakia, which can cause visual impairment.

12.2 CATARACT

Etiologies of cataracts are variable, including aging, genetic, local nutrition obstacles, immunity and *metabolic* abnormality, *trauma*, poisoning, and *radiation*, which all can cause lens metabolism disorders, bring about lens *protein denaturation*, and render the lens turbid. Cataracts are most common in people over 40 years of age, with an incidence that increases with age.

12.2.1 Etiology and Pathogenesis of Cataract

Aging is the most common cause of cataracts. Other common causes and risk factors include *ultraviolet*, smoking, and uncontrolled diabetes. Less common causes are medications, such as corticosteroids, injuries to the eye, and some may even have congenital cataracts due to genetic causes. Cataracts often develop slowly, manifesting with a gradual decline in vision that cannot be corrected by glasses wear. Many degenerative processes *denature* and *coagulate* lens proteins present in lens fibers by different mechanisms, which result in a loss of transparency and, ultimately, cataract formation. There is no medical treatment to prevent the development or progression of cataracts.

12.2.2 Classification

There are different types of cataracts. They may be classified based on the following.

① Etiological: Age-related, traumatic, secondary, metabolic, *toxic*, radiational, developmental cataract, and *posterior capsular opacification*.

② Hereditary: Congenital and acquired cataract.

③ *Morphology* of *opacity*: Punctate, coronary, and perinuclear cataract.

④ Location of opacity: *Cortical*, *nuclear*, posterior *subcapsular*, and mixed cataract (*Figure 12-1*).

⑤ Maturity: Immature, mature, *intumescent*, and hyper-mature cataract.

12.2.3 Clinical Manifestation
12.2.3.1 Symptoms

① Loss of vision.

② Contrast sensitivity reduction: Typically, loss of contrast sensitivity in patients with cataracts has been reported to be greater at higher spatial frequencies. All cataracts lower contrast sensitivity, with posterior subcapsular opacities reported to cause the most significant visual impairment.

③ Refractive power change: Nuclear changes induce a modification of the refractive index of the lens and produce a myopic shift that may be of several diopters or greater. The natural aging of the human lens produces a progressive hyperopic shift.

④ Monocular diplopia: Monocular diplopia is common in patients who have lens opacities, particularly cortical spoke cataracts, which occurs due to a difference when light shines through the water clefts that form these radial wedge shapes and contains a fluid of lower refractive index than the surrounding lens.

⑤ Glare: Even minor degrees of lens opacity cause glare because of a forward scatter of light.

⑥ Color shift: The cataractous lens becomes more absorbent of light towards the blue end of the spectrum, especially with nuclear opacities. Usually, patients are unaware of this color vision defect, but it becomes evident retrospectively after cataract surgery and visual rehabilitation.

⑦ Visual field loss: Depending on the cataract morphology, density, and the location of the opacities, the field of vision may be affected.

12.2.3.2 Signs

Visual acuity is reduced. A slit-lamp examination allows the cataract to be examined in detail and the exact site of any opacity involving the lens can be identified.

12.2.3.3 The lens opacities classification system

The Lens Opacities Classification System Ⅱ (LOCS Ⅱ) has been used in epidemiology studies of the natural history of age-related cataracts. It is a simple classification system based on a set of standardized color photographic transparencies comprising cortical cataract (C), nuclear opalescence (NO), posterior subcapsular cataract (P), and nuclear color (NC), which can be used as a reference to classify lens opacities during the slit-lamp exam or using standardized lens photographs (*Table 12-1*).

Table 12-1 Grades of the lens opacities classification system Ⅱ (LOCS Ⅱ)

Location	Opacities	Label
Nuclear	transparent, distinguish the embryonal nuclei	N0
	early degree of nuclear opalescence	N1
	moderately advanced nuclear opacification	N2
	advanced nuclear opalescence and browning	N3
Cortical	transparent	C0
	a minimal degree of cortical flecking	Ctr
	flecking expansion inside the pupillary margin	C1
	minispokes more than two full quadrants	C2
	obscures approximately 50% of the intrapupillary zone	C3
	obscures approximately 90% of the intrapupillary zone	C4
	obscures more than C4	C5

(To be continued)

(Continued)

Location	Opacities	Label
Posterior	transparent	P0
Subcapsular	filling approximately 3% of the area	P1
	filling approximately 30% of the area	P2
	filling approximately 50% of the area	P3
	more than P3	P4

12.2.3.4 Nuclear sclerosis grading (Emery-Little classification)

An accurate evaluation of lens nucleus hardness is the key to the selection of indications and surgical methods for *phacoemulsification*. The Emery-Little classification was proposed for grading the hardness of nuclear cataracts. Cataracts can be graded by the color of the nucleus after dilation of the pupil (*Table 12-2*).

Table 12-2 Grades of the lens nuclear hardness with the Emery-Little classification

Classification	Medicine name	Lens nuclear color	Label
Grade I	Very soft nuclear	Transparent and nonnuclear	1
Grade II	Soft nuclear	Yellow or yellow-white	2
Grade III	Medium hard nuclear	Dark yellow	3
Grade IV	Hard nuclear	Brown or amber	4
Grade V	Extremely hard nuclear	Dark brown or black	5

12.2.4 Congenital and Developmental Cataract
12.2.4.1 Definition

Congenital and developmental cataracts occur due to some disturbance in the normal growth of the lens. When the disturbance occurs before birth, the child is born with a congenital cataract. Therefore, in congenital cataracts, the opacity is limited to either the embryonic or fetal nucleus. Developmental cataracts may occur from infancy to adolescence. Therefore, such opacities may involve the infantile or adult nucleus, deeper parts of the cortex, or capsule. Developmental cataracts typically affect the particular zone, which is being formed when this process is disturbed. The fibers laid down previously and subsequently are often normally formed and remain transparent. Congenital and developmental opacities may assume the most variable appearances, with minute opacities (those without visual disturbance) being very common in the normal population. These are detectable during slit lamp exams under full mydriasis.

12.2.4.2 Etiology

The exact etiology is not known. Some factors that have been associated with certain types of cataracts are described below.

1) Heredity

Genetically determined cataracts are due to an anomaly in the *chromosomal* pattern of the individual. About one-third of all congenital cataracts are hereditary. The mode of inheritance is usually autosomal dominant. Common familial cataracts include pulverulent cataracts, zonular cataracts (also occur as non-familial), coronary cataracts, and total soft cataracts (may also occur due to *rubella*).

2) Maternal factors

- *Malnutrition* during pregnancy: Malnutrition during pregnancy has been associated with non-familial zonular cataracts.
- Infections: Maternal infections, like rubella, are associated with cataracts in 50% of cases. Other maternal infections associated with congenital cataracts include *toxoplasmosis* and cytomegalic-inclusion disease.
- Drugs ingestion: Congenital cataracts have also been reported in the children of mothers who have taken certain drugs during pregnancy (e.g., thalidomide, corticosteroids).
- Radiation: Maternal exposure to radiation during pregnancy may cause congenital cataracts.

3) Fetal or infantile factors

- Deficient *oxygenation (anoxia)* owing to placental hemorrhage.
- Metabolic disorders of the fetus or infant such as *galactosemia, galactokinase* deficiency, and neonatal *hypoglycemia*.
- Cataracts are associated with other congenital anomalies, e.g. as seen in Lowe's syndrome, *myotonic dystrophy*, and *congenital ichthyosis*.
- Birth trauma.
- Malnutrition in early infancy may also cause developmental cataracts.

4) Idiopathic

About 50% of cases are sporadic and of unknown etiology.

12.2.4.3 Clinical features

Congenital cataracts can occur in one or both eyes. Most are static, but a few continue to develop after birth. Generally, the clinical manifestations are different according to the location, shape, and degree of lens opacity. The common subtypes are capsular, *membranous*, nuclear, *circumnuclear*, anterior polar, posterior polar, blue dot, Coppock, sutural, axial, *coralliform*, floriform, spear-shaped, hard nucleus liquefaction, and total congenital cataract (*Figure 12-2, Figure 12-3*).

12.2.4.4 Evaluation

The diagnosis can be made based on the medical history and the opacity of the lens. When congenital cataracts are combined with malformations of other systems, some laboratory tests should be selected for different situations. Diabetes and neonatal hypoglycemia should be checked for blood sugar, urine sugar, and ketones. Patients with nephropathy should check their urine routine and urine amino acids. Patients with suspected metabolic disease should be tested for blood amino acid levels. In addition, urine phenylpyruvate determination, qualitative examination of homocystinuria, and screening of galactosemia can be checked.

12.2.4.5 Management

1) Clinic-investigative workup

A detailed clinical investigative workup is paramount in the management of *pediatric* cataracts. It should aim towards knowing the prognostic factors and indications, as well as the ideal timing of surgery.

① Ocular examination should be carried out with special reference to:
- Density and morphology of cataract.
- Assessment of visual function is difficult in infants and small children. The density and morphology of the cataract may be elucidated by oblique illumination examination and fundus examination. Special tests, like fixation reflex, forced-choice preferential looking test, visually evoked potential (VEP), optic-kinetic nystagmus (OKN), etc., also provide useful information.
- Associated ocular defects should be noted, such as microphthalmos, glaucoma, PHPV, foveal hypoplasia, optic nerve hypoplasia, rubella retinopathy, etc.

② Laboratory investigations should be carried out to detect the following systemic associations in non-hereditary cataracts:
- Intrauterine infections. Particularly, toxoplasmosis, rubella, cytomegalovirus, and herpes virus by TORCH testing.
- Galactosemia via a urine test for reducing substances, red blood cell transferase, and galactokinase levels.
- Lowe's syndrome via urine chromatography for amino acids.
- Hyperglycemia via blood sugar.
- Hypocalcemia via serum calcium and phosphate levels and X-ray skull.

2) Prognostic factors which need to be noted
- Density of cataract.
- Unilateral or bilateral cataract.
- Time of presentation.
- Associated ocular defects.
- Associated systemic defects.

3) Indications and timing of pediatric cataract surgery
- Partial cataracts and small central cataracts that are visually insignificant can safely be ignored and observed or may need non-surgical treatment with pupillary

dilatation.
- For unilateral or binocular cataracts or cataracts located in the center of the optic axis with obvious opacity, surgery should be performed as soon as possible after birth, no later than 6 months. Other surgeries should be performed as soon as possible after the completion of one operation.
- Unilateral dense cataracts should preferably be removed as early as possible after birth. However, it must be borne in mind that visual *prognosis* in most unilateral cases is very poor even after the timely operation because correction of aphakia and prevention of amblyopia in infants is an uphill task.

4) Surgical procedures
- Childhood cataracts (congenital, developmental as well as acquired) can be dealt with via anterior *capsulotomy* and aspiration of the lens or *lensectomy*.
- Note: Needling operation (which was performed in the past) is now obsolete.

5) Correction of pediatric aphakia

This is still an unsolved problem. Presently common views are as follows:
- Children above the age of 2 years can be corrected with the implantation of an intraocular lens during surgery.
- Children below the age of 2 years should preferably be treated using extended-wear contact lenses. Spectacles can be prescribed in bilateral cataract cases. Later on, secondary IOL implantation may be considered. The present trend is to do primary implantation at the earliest possible time (within 2~3 months), especially in unilateral cataract cases.

6) Pediatric IOL: size, design, and refractive power

The main concerns regarding the use of IOL in children include the growth of the eye, IOL power considerations, increased uveal reaction and long-term safety. Present recommendations are :
- Size of IOL above the age of 2 years may be standard 12 to 12.75 mm diameter for in the bag implantation.
- The design of IOL recommended is one-piece PMMA with modified C-shaped haptics (preferably heparin coated).
- Refractive power of IOL. In children between 2~8 years of age, 10% under-correction from the calculated biometric power is recommended to counter the myopic shift. Below two years of under-correction by 20% is recommended.

12.2.5 Acquired Cataract
12.2.5.1 Definition

In general, any factor, physical, chemical, or biological, that disturbs the critical intra and extracellular equilibrium of water and electrolytes or deranges the colloid system within the lens fibers tends to bring about opacification.

12.2.5.2 Etiology

Cataracts are typically classified by location.

① Cortical cataracts: Cortical cataracts are caused by swelling, degeneration, and liquefaction of the younger outer (cortical) fibers. It is commonly seen in age-related cataracts and can be subdivided into four consecutive stages as the cataract progresses.

- Incipient stage: The lens appears as a vacuole or water gap within the cortex and is typified by a cuneiform opacification pointed towards the center (*Figure 12-4*). With associated slow progression, this subtype does not influence visual acuity significantly.

- Intumescent stage: Otherwise known as immature stage, impaired vision is often detected as the opacification of the lens aggravates. When examined under oblique illumination, a crescent-shaped shadow can be detected within the pupillary zone, the characteristic "iris shadow" (*Figure 12-5*). With the absorption of water, the inflated and enlarged lens pushes the iris plane towards the cornea, resulting in a shallow anterior chamber. Acute angle-closure glaucoma may be induced with a predisposed anatomical basis.

- Mature stage: With total milky opacity of the lens (*Figure 12-6*), the visual acuity of the patient can decrease due to hand movement (HM) or light perception(LP), and the fundus is usually not visible. As fluids exude from the capsule, the shape of the lens shrinks back, accompanied by a recovered depth of the anterior chamber. The iris shadow may not be detectable anymore in this subtype.

- Hypermature stage: The further shrunken lens and wrinkled capsule caused by lens fiber liquefaction make the anterior chamber deeper. Consequently, iridodonesis can be revealed. The nucleus floats freely within the capsule (Morgagnian cataract) (*Figure 12-7*). The potential complications induced by the outflowed cortex include phaco anaphylactic uveitis and phacolytic glaucoma.

② Nuclear sclerotic cataracts: Nuclear sclerotic cataracts are due to diffuse lens hardening and discoloration (yellow, green, white, or brown) from deterioration of the older central (nuclear) fibers. This increases the index of refraction, often resulting in a myopic shift, commonly known as "second sight", in presbyopic individuals who are once again able to read without glasses when their cataract progresses. Eventually, however, the second sight is overshadowed by the decreased vision from the cataract. Extreme nuclear sclerosis may produce a dark mahogany-colored, almost black lens (cataract nigrans).

③ Subcapsular cataracts: Subcapsular cataracts occur just beneath the lens capsule.

- Anterior subcapsular cataract (ASC) : Fibrous plaque from metaplasia of the central anterior lens epithelial cells.

- Posterior subcapsular cataract (PSC) : Granular opacity from posterior migration and swelling of epithelial cells.

Cataracts may also be categorized by etiology.

① Age-related cataracts: All forms of cataracts are most commonly due to aging changes involving environmental factors, metabolism, nutritional status, and hereditary background as the potential underlying mechanism. Additional risk factors may include aging, female gender, smoking, alcohol abuse, trauma, diabetes mellitus, hypertension, etc.

② Systemic diseases associated with cataracts: Systemic diseases can produce characteristic cataracts, e.g. diabetic cataract (cortical or PSC cataract), galactose cataract (perinuclear cataract), hypocalcemia, also called tetany cataract (white dots or flakes in the lens), myotonic dystrophy (central, polychromatic, iridescent, cortical crystals that have the appearance of a "Christmas tree"), Wilson's disease ["sun-flower cataract"(chalcosis lentis)], Fabry's disease, atopic dermatitis (PSC cataract), neurofibromatosis type 2 (PSC cataract), and ectodermal dysplasia.

③ Eye disease associated cataracts: Also known as complicated cataract secondary to uveitis (ASC or PSC cataract), angle-closure glaucoma (glaukomflecken), intraocular tumors (sector cataract near the tumor), retinitis pigmentosa (PSC cataract), Stickler's syndrome (cortical cataract).

④ Toxic cataracts: Medications are the primary cause of toxic cataracts and include steroids (PSC cataract), miotics (ASC cataract), phenothiazines (ASC cataract), amiodarone (ASC cataract), and busulfan (PSC cataract). Toxic cataract also result from radiation [ionizing (PSC cataract), infrared (anterior capsule exfoliation), ultraviolet, argon laser (nuclear sclerotic cataract), microwave, and short-wave], electricity (cortical cataract), and chemicals (i.e. mercury).

⑤ Traumatic cataracts: Blunt trauma often results in a cortical rosette-pattern cataract, penetrating trauma leads to a cataract if the lens capsule is perforated due to hydration of the lens, and an intraocular foreign body can produce a distinctive cataract if it contains iron (orange ASC deposits) or copper (green lens capsule and cortical petaloid pattern).

⑥ Postoperative cataracts: After almost any intraocular surgery, there is an increased risk of cataracts. This is especially true if silicon oil is used in retinal surgery.

12.2.5.3 Clinical features

With early cataracts, vision may be unchanged. Over time, patients experience painless progressive blurring of vision, dimmer vision with the need for more light to see clearly, glare from bright light sources, and occasionally monocular diplopia. If left untreated, cataracts can lead to blindness.

12.2.5.4 Evaluation

Medical history taking should include screening for any systemic diseases, medications (especially prior use of steroids), ocular trauma or surgery, radiation exposure, and other ocular diseases. It is also important to characterize the patient's visual changes, inquire about the functional difficulties they cause, and note any exacerbating factors (e.g. near versus distance, at night, with bright lights).

A complete eye exam is performed and should concentrate on quantifying the decreased vision (distance and near acuity, pinhole, refraction, glare testing, contrast sensitivity, and color vision) and documenting the appearance of the cataract (type, size, density, and location). It is important to rule out other causes of poor vision, so attention must also be directed to the cornea (for central staining, edema, or scarring), tonometry (for increased IOP), gonioscopy, and ophthalmoscopy (for macular pathology). B-scan ultrasonography should be performed to ensure no posterior segment problems if the fundus cannot be adequately visualized through the cataract. Keratometry and A-scan biometry must be performed to calculate the intraocular lens (IOL) implant power before cataract surgery. Advanced instruments, including IOL-master (Zeiss, Oberkochen, Germany) or Lenstar LS900 (Haag-Streit, Koniz, Switzerland), can be optional for the calculation of lens power.

12.2.5.5 Management

The only way to restore vision is the surgical removal of the cloudy lens with IOL implantation. The indications for cataract extraction and insertion of an IOL are: visual symptoms interfere with specific activities, and the patient desires improved visual function, a cataract that causes other ocular diseases (e.g., secondary glaucoma or uveitis), or a cataract that prevents adequate examination or treatment of a pre-existing posterior-segment condition (e.g., diabetic retinopathy, age-related macular degeneration, or glaucoma).

Cataract surgery has undergone dramatic evolution during the past 30 years, developing from the original intracapsular cataract extraction (ICCE) to the extracapsular cataract extraction (ECCE), to the currently performed phacoemulsification. All this has occurred alongside the introduction of the operating microscope and microsurgical instruments, improving the development of intraocular lenses, the alterations in techniques, and local *anesthesia*. The duration of the surgery has also decreased while the postoperative prognosis has improved. Currently, phacoemulsification with foldable IOL implantation is the predominant surgery for cataracts. The recently introduced femtosecond laser-assisted cataract surgery will hopefully further reduce the risk of intraoperative and postoperative complications.

12.2.6 Posterior Capsular Opacification
12.2.6.1 Definition

Posterior capsular opacification (PCO) refers to a clouding of the normally clear posterior lens capsule after cataract surgery.

12.2.6.2 Etiology

PCO is due to the proliferation, migration, and epithelial-mesenchymal transition of residual lens epithelial cells along the posterior capsule, leading to capsular fibrosis. PCO is sometimes referred to as a secondary cataract since the vision becomes decreased and symptoms of a cataract return again after successful cataract surgery. PCO has different components based on formation mechanism and morphology.

① Soemmering ring: The remaining equatorial lens epithelial cells continue to proliferate and produce new cortical fibers that, over time, progress to form a ring between the posterior capsule and the edges of the anterior capsule remnant.

② Elschnig pearl: This typical form of regeneratory PCO develops gradually, first forming syncytial and later clustered peals.

③ Fibrotic PCO: This subtype is caused by transdifferentiated LECs from the anterior capsule that gain access to the posterior capsule and cause whitening and wrinkling of the capsule.

④ Mixed form of regeneratory and fibrotic PCO.

12.2.6.3 Clinical features

① Symptoms: Mild PCO is usually asymptomatic. The symptoms of a significant PCO are decreased vision, glare, or streaks radiating from lights.

② Signs: PCO is evident on slit-lamp examination as whitening and/or wrinkling of the posterior capsule, usually best appreciated with the pupil dilated (*Figure 12-8*).

12.2.6.4 Evaluation

Patient history should be documented when the previous cataract surgery was performed.

A comprehensive eye exam must be done with particular attention to the vision (distance and near acuity, pin-hole, refraction) and posterior capsule (size, density, and location of the opacity). It is also necessary to rule out other causes of decreased vision with careful inspection of the cornea (for central staining, edema, or scarring), IOL (presence, position, and stability), and ophthalmoscopy (for macular pathology).

12.2.6.5 Management

The definitive treatment for a visually significant PCO involves creating a central opening in the capsule (posterior capsulotomy). This is accomplished by using a Nd: YAG laser with a slit-lamp delivery system (*Figure 12-9*). Surgical membranes may be a differential for a thick opacity.

12.3 MANAGEMENT OF CATARACT

12.3.1 Surgical Indications and Surgical Contraindications

① Surgical indications: In the past, a mature staged cataract was considered the best surgical period. Now, due to the advancement of surgical technology and medical equipment, it is generally believed that surgery can be performed when the visual function no longer meets the needs of the patient. Cataract removal is also suitable when lens opacity hinders the best treatment of posterior segment diseases and when the lens causes inflammation (phacolysis, lens *allergic* reaction), anterior chamber angle closure, and angle-closure glaucoma that cannot be controlled by drugs.

In addition, a doctor must consider the following questions before deciding on an operation: a. Whether the degree of lens opacity is consistent with the degree of vision loss of the patient; b. Whether the lens opacity is secondary to other systems or eye diseases; c. Whether the patient can achieve an ideal visual acuity postoperatively. To answer the above questions, detailed preoperative inspections and preparations are required.

② Surgical contraindications: For patients with diabetes, high blood pressure, heart failure, lung infection, and other serious systemic diseases that are not suitable for surgery, the surgeon must always ask the internal medicine department to strictly control these before considering surgery. For patients with other comorbid eye diseases, including chronic dacryocystitis, eyelid inversion or ectropion, trichiasis, active inflammation of the ocular surface such as keratitis, acute bacterial conjunctivitis, viral or fungal keratitis, or other intraocular inflammation, such as uveitis, they are not immediately suitable for cataract surgery.

12.3.2 Preoperative Examination

① The systemic preoperative examination for cataract surgery includes heart, lung, liver, and kidney function examination to ensure that the patient can tolerate the operation; if necessary, consult with the internal medicine department. Hypertensive or diabetic patients need blood pressure and blood sugar control, as well as coagulation function examinations. Hepatitis B, syphilis, and other infectious diseases screening is needed.

② Ocular examination pre-cataract surgery includes vision, corrected vision, intraocular pressure, red and green perception; silt lamp, ophthalmoscope examination, recording the degree of the cornea, iris, anterior chamber, and lens opacity. Furthermore, checking the vitreous body after mydriasis, retina, macula, and optic nerve, as well as excluding active ocular inflammation and fundus disease.

③ Examination of eye appendages includes eyelids, lacrimal organs, conjunctiva, eye position and eye movement, and orbit, which are very important for the safety and quality of cataract surgery.

④ Special examinations include intraocular pressure, corneal curvature, axial length measurement, calculation of intraocular lens power, corneal topography, corneal endothelial cells, ocular B-ultrasound, comprehensive ocular surface analysis, optical quality analysis, and other inspections.

- The accuracy of biological eye measurement before cataract surgery directly determines the accuracy of intraocular lens calculation and significantly affects the refractive state and surgical effect after cataract surgery. At present, the preoperative biological measurement of cataracts mainly includes corneal curvature measurement and axial length measurement.

- At present, there are three main methods for clinical corneal curvature measurement: keratometer method, optical detection method (optical coherence biometer IOLmaster, Lenstar, etc.), and corneal topography method (Orbscan; Bausch and Lomb, Laval, Canada, Pentacam; Oculus Inc., Arlinglton, WA, USA, etc.). When measuring the corneal curvature by the above three different methods, the keratometer and IOLmaster corneal curvature measurement range is about 4 mm in the central cornea. However, it can only measure the curvature radius of the anterior corneal surface but not the individualized posterior corneal refractive power and its astigmatism. Based on the data of the anterior surface of the cornea, without considering the posterior surface of the cornea, there will be measurement errors in the pathological and irregular cornea, and it is hard to find keratoconus. In addition, the total corneal refractive power obtained by IOLmaster is a simulated corneal refractive power, which cannot truly reflect the refractive state of the entire cornea. The automatic keratometer can be examined in a lying position, which is more convenient for children or patients in general anesthesia. The corneal topography allows the surgeon to fully understand the refractive condition of the entire cornea. Corneal topography (Orbscan, Pentacam, etc.) should be examined before cataract surgery for patients who wish to have multifocal IOLS implanted (*Figure 12-10*).

- The axial length refers to the distance from the corneal vertex to the fovea of the macula. Studies found that 54% of the refractive error after cataract surgery comes from the measurement error of the axial length, which indicates that the measurement of the axial length is the focus before cataract surgery. Based on different principles and technologies, there are two types of axial measurement: acoustic instrument measurement (A-mode ultrasound) and optical instrument measurement (IOLmaster, Lenster, etc.). With the advent of optical measuring instruments, optical measurements with better accuracy, portability, repeatability, and non-contact have begun to be used in clinical applications and continue to be promoted. The newly launched IOLmaster700 (Zeiss, Oberkochen, Germany) uses the sweep frequency technique, which has stronger penetrating power and a higher detection rate than the IOLmaster500 (Zeiss, Oberkochen, Germany). However, for patients with severe cataracts, poor fixation, nystagmus, and low-cooperation, optical measurement is often difficult to proceed with or inaccurate (*Figure 12-11*).

- Corneal endothelial examination before cataract surgery mainly includes the number, morphology, and average area of corneal endothelial cells. The main content of the preoperative examination is the density of corneal endothelial cells (CD: pcs/mm^2), the shape, and the ratio of hexagonal cells (%). According to age changes, the average density of normal corneal endothelium decreases, and the proportion of hexagonal cells decreases. For patients with an average corneal endothelial density lower than 1000/mm^2, cataract surgery should be carefully considered to avoid postoperative corneal endothelial decompensation, which will affect the surgical effect (*Figure 12-12*).

- Studies have found that cataract surgery can affect the normal physiological function of the ocular surface and tear film of the operated eye, accelerate the evaporation of tears, reduce the quality of tears, and even lead to dry eyes, that is, post-cataract surgery dry eye. Therefore, for cataract patients, ocular surface and tear film examinations should be performed before surgery, and routine inspections for dry eyes should be performed simultaneously. This is especially important for patients who require higher visual quality after surgery. In recent years, a comprehensive ocular surface analyzer (Keratograph; Oculus Inc, Arlington, WA, USA) for systematic examination of the ocular surface and dry eye can record the tear river height, breakup time, tear film quality, meibomian gland function, etc., and systematically evaluate the health of the patient's ocular surface state, to provide a good visual quality and quality of life after surgery (*Figure 12-13*).

- For some cataract patients, it is hard to check the fundus. B-ultrasound can observe the intraocular conditions of the posterior segment of the eye, including the vitreous body, retina, and optic nerve.

- For the selection of multifocal intraocular lenses and Toric intraocular lenses, the estimation of visual quality before surgery, corneal spherical aberration, high-order corneal aberration, pupil diameter, Kappa angle, and corneal astigmatism are also important guiding roles. Therefore, some emerging optical inspection instruments, such as Pentacam and OPD examination parameters have further reference values (*Figure 12-14*). OPD: Zernike images, PSF images, MTF images, and visual simulation images can further intuitively evaluate the visual quality after cataract surgery. With better accuracy, repetitive inspections, this item has begun to be used in clinical applications and continues to be promoted.

⑤ Vision prediction after cataract surgery: decreased vision is the main reason for cataract patients to seek medical treatment, so vision prediction after cataract surgery is essential. Because the cloudy lens prevents direct observation of the retina, some methods must be taken to evaluate the function of the retina and macula. Meanwhile, some emerging optical instruments can provide visual quality-related information and provide a more intuitive and detailed preview of the postoperative effect.

- Visual electrophysiology examination: Electrophysiology includes electroretinogram (ERG) examination and visual evoked potential (VEP) examination. ERG examination reflects the function of retinal cone cells, rod cells, and mixed functions. Retinitis pigmentosa, retinal circulation disorders, retinal detachment, and other retinal diseases patients are of obvious abnormalities. VEP is a cluster of electrical signals generated by the occipital area of the brain to visual stimuli, representing the transmission of visual information above the optic ganglion cells. It is generally considered to be an objective visual examination method. In patients with macular degeneration, glaucoma, and optic nerve disease, VEP can be significantly abnormal.

- Optical coherence tomography: Due to the development of optical instruments, the resolution of the instrument and the depth of tissue penetration have significantly improved. For patients whose lenses are not completely cloudy, the macular area of the retina can be observed through OCT, further to evaluate the function of the macular area so as to have a certain estimate of postoperative visual acuity.

12.3.3 Phacoemulsification

The following are the steps for phacoemulsification:

① *Levofloxacin* or *tobramycin* or gentamicin three times a day for three days pre-operatively in order to prevent intraocular infection.

② Irrigation of conjunctival sac and *lacrimal ducts* using 0.9% saline before the operation to protect against *endophthalmitis*.

③ Compound tropicamide eye drops are used every 15 minutes at least three times in one hour before surgery to dilate the pupil adequately.

④ Local anesthesia is preferred for cataract surgery via *proparacaine hydrochloride*, *oxybuprocaine* hydrochloride eye drops, peri-, or retrobulbar injection of *lidocaine*, or in combined use for the operation. For special patients, like children or adults who cannot tolerate the surgery, phacoemulsification may be performed under general anesthesia.

⑤ After aseptic preparation and laying a sterile plastic drape to open the lids and expose the operative eye, the lids are retracted using a lid speculum.

⑥ Retract lids using a lid speculum.

⑦ *Corneoscleral* incision required is very small (3 mm), which enables suture-less surgery with a self-sealing scleral tunnel or clear corneal incision. *Continuous curvilinear capsulorrhexis (CCC)* of 4~6 mm is preferred over other methods of anterior capsulotomy. Hydrodissection, i.e. separation of the capsule from the cortex by injecting fluid exactly between the two is a must for phacoemulsification in SICS. This procedure facilitates nucleus rotation and manipulation during phacoemulsification. Nucleus is emulsified and aspirated by phacoemulsifier. Phacoemulsifier basically acts through a hollow 1 mm titanium needle, which vibrates courtesy of a piezoelectric crystal along its longitudinal axis at an ultrasonic speed of 40 000 times a second and thus emulsifies the nucleus. Many different techniques are being used to accomplish phacoemulsification. Remaining cortical lens matter is aspirated with the help of an irrigation-aspiration technique. IOL implantation, removal of *viscoelastic* substance, and wound closure. A foldable IOL is most ideal with the phacoemulsification technique. (*Figure 12-15*)

12.3.4 Intraocular Lens Options

① Aspheric intraocular lenses: An optimized surface curvature to correct the higher-order aberration of the spherical aberration, contrast sensitivity, especially for large pupils.

② Toric intraocular lenses: If the patient's corneal astigmatism is greater than 1.0 D, toric IOL compensates with a corresponding optical zone.

③ Multifocal intraocular lenses: Multifocal lenses enable near and distant vision by giving two or more focal points to get better vision, including refractive lenses, diffractive lenses, and lenses combing diffractive and refractive optics.

④ Accommodative intraocular lenses: Accommodative lenses have restored accommodative focus and adapted to anteroposterior lens displacement. However, this type of IOL is still under development and in the testing phase.

⑤ Blue light-filtering ("yellow") intraocular lenses: Blue light-filtering ("yellow") intraocular lenses reduce the transmission of short-wave light to get less injury of photo-oxidative injury of the retina, without impairing contrast vision.

12.3.5 Complications of Cataract Surgery and Management

① Local anesthesia complications: Retrobulbar hemorrhage, perforation of the globe, and allergic reactions, like hypotension, and respiratory paralysis. Topical anesthesia markedly reduces these complications, especially for patients taking anticoagulants.

② Prolapse of uveal tissue through the surgical entry wound: Viscoelastic protection may reduce damage to the iris by surgical instruments.

③ Corneal injury, such as separation of Descemet's membrane or corneal thermal injury from the phacoemulsification tip is dealt with via eliminating causes and use of medical agents to reduce intraoperative injury of cornea.

④ Tearing of the lens capsular sac with *subluxation* of the IOL, incarceration, or loss of the vitreous body: Familiarity with capsulotomy and nuclear fragmentation reduces the chance of breaking the posterior capsule. However, once the tearing of the capsular sac and incarceration of the vitreous has occurred, the operator must be more careful to deal with the residual nucleus or cortex. A vitrectomy may be performed to remove the vitreous body within the anterior chamber. Intraocular lens implantation may be delayed.

⑤ Severe hemorrhage, like choroidal effusion, or expulsive hemorrhage: These are really rare. Once this happens though, one must dose close all incision(s) immediately, use intravenous medications to make the patient calm down, and lower IOP. Safer surgery may be conducted once with no more bleeding and controlled IOP.

⑥ Pain may be due to injury of the corneal epithelium: Lubricants and soft contact lens can treat these pains.

⑦ Endophthalmitis: A rare complication. Strict antiseptic precautions can markedly reduce endophthalmitis rates. Once endophthalmitis does arise, medical and/or surgical treatment should be provided as rapidly and as soon as possible.

⑧ *Cystoid macular edema*: May occur 1~3 months after cataract surgery and usually regresses in a further six months, and some patients progress towards a macular hole. Preoperative evaluation of the fundus and regular examinations of the retina postoperatively are necessary for every cataract patient in order to treat macular diseases immediately and help in visual rehabilitation.

⑨ Rhegmatogenous retinal detachment: 1%~2% of patients would suffer this within one year following cataract surgery. During this period, patients need to have regular dilated fundus examination, retinal laser coagulation, or surgery if necessary.

⑩ Glaucoma: Firstly, the surgeon must determine the cause of any IOP elevation that develops after surgery. Topical and systemic medicine, conventional laser treatment, and surgery for glaucoma may be required for IOP control, depending on the specific etiology.

⑪ Postoperative cataract: Treated via laser capsulotomy with a *neodymium*-YAG laser.

12.4 DISLOCATED LENS (ECTOPIA LENTIS)

12.4.1 Definition

Ectopia lentis refers to a dislocation or displacement of the natural crystalline lens from its normal position, centered behind the iris. It is usually bilateral, symmetric, and non-progressive. In *lens subluxation*, the lens is partially dislocated but remains in the pupillary aperture with incomplete disruption of lens zonule fibers. In *lens luxation* (dislocation), the lens is completely detached from the ciliary body. Luxated lenses may dislocate into either the anterior or posterior chamber due to the complete separation of lens zonule fibers.

12.4.2 Etiology

The most common cause of acquired lens displacement is trauma. Traumatic ectopia lentis is most often the result of direct damage to the eye, but can also occur after blunt trauma to the head or orbit.

Ectopia lentis can also occur due to ocular disease or systemic disease. More commonly, lens displacement is associated with systemic syndromes, such as Marfan syndrome, homocystinuria, and Weill-Marchesani syndrome. It can also be associated with other ocular disorders such as congenital disorder or as a spontaneous disorder, aniridia, pseudoexfoliation syndrome, and congenital glaucoma.

Other less common conditions associated with ectopia lentis include Ehlers-Danlos syndrome, sulfite oxidase deficiency, hyperlysinemia, congenital syphilis, Apert's disease, ectopia lentis et pupillae, *spherophakia*, iris *coloboma*, retinitis pigmentosa, intraocular tumor, Reiger syndrome, megalocornea, hypermature cataract, high Myopia, buphthalmos, and anterior uveal tumors.

12.4.3 Lens Subluxation

Lens Subluxation may vary from an asymptomatic mild displacement, seen only in post-pupillary dilation, to a significant subluxation that places the equator of the lens in the pupillary axis. Clinical features are as follows:

① Red painful eye (secondary to trauma).

② Marked astigmatism.

③ Lenticular myopia.

④ Decreased vision.

⑤ Monocular diplopia.

⑥ Portion of the lens presents in the pupillary area.

⑦ Deep and irregular anterior chamber.

Chapter 12 Lens Diseases

⑧ Iridodenesis (tremulous iris).
⑨ Floaters.
⑩ Raised intraocular pressure when aqueous flow is blocked.
⑪ Slit lamp: edge of subluxated lens can be seen in a dilated pupil (*Figure 12-16*).

12.4.4 Lens Luxation
12.4.4.1 Classification
① Anterior luxation: The lens dislocates into the pupil or the anterior chamber, and physically pushes the iris posteriorly. A forward dislocation of the lens may cause pupillary block with the subsequent development of acute glaucoma or chronic closed-angle glaucoma, leading to corneal edema. A dislocated lens can also cause a focal area of corneal endothelial edema by direct touch of the corneal endothelium.

② Posterior luxation: The lens falls backward behind the iris and dislocates into the vitreous, leading to aphakia in the pupillary exam and iridodonesis. When the lens is luxated, the depth of the anterior chamber will usually increase, regardless of the direction of the luxation. A posterior lens luxation may cause vitreous traction on the retina, leading to uveitis, chronic vitritis, chorioretinal inflammation, or retinal detachment.

12.4.4.2 Complications
① Complete dislocation.
② Cataractous changes.
③ Uveitis.
④ Vitreitis.
⑤ Chorioretinal inflammation.
⑥ Secondary glaucoma (Pupillary block glaucoma).
⑦ Corneal endothelial cell damage and corneal endothelial edema.
⑧ Vitreous hemorrhage.
⑨ Hyphema.
⑩ Retinal detachment.
⑪ Globe rupture.

12.4.4.3 Diagnosis/Evaluation
① History.
- History of any recent trauma.
- History of associated ocular and systemic diseases.

② Physical examination.
- Visual acuity.
- Slit lamp exam.
- Retinoscopy and refraction.
- Dilated fundus examination.
- Ultrasound (lens displaced from usual position, evidence of other associated

traumatic injuries).
- Corneal diameter (megalocornea).
- Intraocular pressure.
- Keratometry.

③ Laboratory tests.
- Total plasma homocysteine concentration (Homocystinuria).
- Cardiac evaluation (Marfan syndrome).
- Other hereditary conditions.

12.4.4.4 Management

① Non-surgical.
- Genetic counseling.
- Optical correction of the refractive error.
- Medically treatment of any elevation in intraocular pressure.
- Progressive lens dislocation without major complications has been traditionally managed conservatively.

② Surgery.

The decision to operate depends on many factors, including visual acuity, lens location, progressive subluxation of the lens, imminent total dislocation, and others. Techniques include:
- Laser peripheral iridotomy for pupillary block glaucoma.
- Lensectomy/vitrectomy with postoperative optical rehabilitation using a contact lens.
- Iris-fixated intraocular lens.
- Scleral-sutured posterior intraocular lens.
- Implantation of in-the-bag intraocular lens with a capsular tension ring.
- *Femtosecond laser technology* can aid in the surgical management of subluxated cataracts.

12.5 CONGENITAL ANOMALIES OF THE LENS

Congenital lens anomalies include abnormalities of lens formation, morphology, transparency, and position, which can occur at different stages from embryonic lens vesicle formation to birth. This section mainly introduces abnormalities of lens formation and morphology.

12.5.1 Abnormal Lens Formation
12.5.1.1 Clinical features

① Congenital aphakia or primary aphakia refers to the absence of a lens placode in the early embryo, and is rarely seen in the clinic. Secondary aphakia is a degenerative change after formation of the lens, resulting in the disappearance of the lens and leaving only traces of its prior existence, combined with microphthalmia and other ocular structure dysplasia.

② Lens agenesis: Corneal opacity, posterior keratoconus, and anterior cone-shaped deformity of lens occur when the separation of lens vesicle and surface ectodermal is delayed in the embryonic period. Hypoplasia of lens fibers may result in binuclear, anuclear, or abnormal fissures within the lens.

12.5.1.2 Evaluation

Slit-lamp examination confirms the diagnosis of abnormal lens formation, depending on the morphology of the observed lens.

12.5.1.3 Management

No special treatment is required.

12.5.2 Abnormal Lens Morphology

12.5.2.1 Clinical features

① Spherophakia: Spherophakia may occur as an isolated familial condition or as a feature of other syndromes, mostly bilateral. The lens is spherical in shape (not normally biconvex) and small in size, which may lead to lens dislocation. When the pupil is fully dilated, the equator and *suspensory* ligament of the lens are completely exposed. Due to the relaxation of the suspensory ligament, the lens moves forward, which tends to cause pupillary block and angle-closure glaucoma. The increase in the refractive power of the spherical lens may lead to high myopia. Due to the extension of the suspensive ligament of the lens, the pulling force is weakened, therefore causing a total loss of accommodation.

② *Lenticonus*: This refers to a cone-shaped elevation of the anterior pole or posterior pole of the lens, usually occurring in the late fetal period or after birth. It is a rare congenital anomaly of the lens, especially the lenticonus anterior, often associated with congenital cataracts and high myopia.

③ Coloboma of the lens: This is usually unilateral and often hereditary. There is a notch-like defect involving the lower quadrant of the equator, with different shapes and sizes. The suspensory ligament is reduced or absent in the defect. The refractive power of the lens is unequal in all directions, with myopic astigmatism.

④ *Umbilication* of the lens: There is a slight depression on the anterior or posterior surface of the lens, which is extremely rare.

12.5.2.2 Evaluation

Slit-lamp examination confirms the diagnosis, depending on the morphology of the observed lens.

12.5.2.3 Management

① Treatment is generally not necessary when there are no symptoms or complications.

② Miotics should not be used in patients with spherophakia.

③ Surgery may be required in cases with lens dislocation and cataracts.

④ Correct amblyopia.

Chapter 13
Retinal Diseases

INTRODUCTION
RETINAL VASCULAR DISEASE
- ▶ Retinal Artery Occlusion (RAO)
- ▶ Retinal Vein Occlusion (RVO)

MACULOPATHY
- ▶ Age-Related Macular Degeneration (AMD)
- ▶ Central Serous Chorioretinopathy (CSC)

RETINITIS PIGMENTOSA (RP)
- ▶ Pathogenesis
- ▶ Symptoms and Clinical Features
- ▶ Differential Diagnosis
- ▶ Treatment/Management
- ▶ Prognosis

SYSTEMIC DISEASES AND RETINOPATHY
- ▶ Hypertensive Retinopathy
- ▶ Diabetic Retinopathy (DR)

RETINAL DETACHMENT (RD)
- ▶ Risk Factors
- ▶ Pathogenesis
- ▶ Symptoms and Clinical Features
- ▶ Treatment/Management
- ▶ Prognosis

13.1 INTRODUCTION

The retina is delicate in structure and complex in function and is susceptible to various pathogenic factors. At the same time, it is susceptible to autovascular diseases and systemic vascular diseases. In this chapter, it is necessary to learn the influence of the special structure and function of the retina on retinopathy, as well as the damage of the retina caused by systemic diseases.

13.2 RETINAL VASCULAR DISEASE

13.2.1 Retinal Artery Occlusion (RAO)

Central retinal artery occlusion (CRAO) is a catastrophic ophthalmic emergency that severely impairs a patient's visual function. It was complete obstruction of the central retinal artery (CRA) leading to retinal *ischemia*, rapidly progressive cellular damage, and vision loss. Retina survival depends on the degree of collateralization and the duration of retinal ischemia. The CRA originates from the ophthalmic artery, which is the first branch of the internal carotid artery. The CRA and its branches supply blood to the inner retina, including the macula and fovea. Occlusion of a branch of the CRA causes a branch retinal artery occlusion(BRAO).

13.2.1.1 Risk factors

RAO and cerebral ischemic stroke share similar risk factors, including systemic *comorbidities* (critical carotid disease, hypertension, tobacco use, hyperlipidemia, cardiac valvular disease, migraine, sickle cell disease, atherosclerosis, aortic disease, aneurysm, diabetes, and carotid and coronary artery diseases). The incidence increases with age. Generally, the incidence is higher in men than in women.

13.2.1.2 Pathogenesis

Any process that obstructs the blood flow to the CRA can cause a CRAO. Similar to *cerebral infarctions* in the anterior circulation, the most common cause of CRAO and BRAO is an *embolus* in the affected artery. Such emboli originate most often from the *ipsilateral internal carotid artery*, followed by the aortic arch, and the heart. The three main types of emboli are *cholesterol*, calcium, and *platelet fibrin*. On *fundus* photography, calcium emboli appear white, cholesterol emboli appear orange, and platelet-fibrin emboli appear dull white.

13.2.1.3 Symptoms and clinical features

Typically, there is a sudden, painless, monocular vision loss that occurs over seconds. It can occur at any time of the day. Patients may report an antecedent transient visual loss and often have a history of *atherosclerotic* disease.

Patients with CRAO often present with monocular loss of light perception and an afferent pupillary defect. Visual acuity can vary from loss of light perception to finger counting.

There are three stages of CRAO: incomplete, subtotal, and total. These stages have the following clinical characteristics. Incomplete CRAO is characterized by reduced visual acuity, an inconspicuous cherry-red spot on the retina, mild retinal edema, and delayed blood flow. Subtotal CRAO is characterized by severely decreased visual acuity, a conspicuous cherry-red spot on the retina, and substantially diminished/interrupted blood flow. Total CRAO differs from subtotal CRAO in that there is no light perception and no blood flow in the perimacular arterioles.

The retinal opacity usually starts to resolve in about a week and generally resolves completely within about a month or so, and the retina regains its transparency.

FFA shows eyes with CRAO display longer CRA perfusion time, compared with normal eyes, as well as incomplete retinal perfusion.

As a non-invasive imaging system, *enhanced depth imaging-assisted optical coherence tomography (EDI-OCT)* allows accurate documentation and staging of CRAO severity, along with a general assessment of the visual outcome. The degrees of inner and outer retinal edema in the acute phase, as well as subsequent thinning of the retina and choroid, can be clearly detected by EDI-OCT.

Optical coherence tomography angiography (OCTA) shows extensive disruption of the superficial and deep capillary plexus is visible, but disruption is greater in the superficial capillary plexus.

13.2.1.4 Differential diagnosis

- Ophthalmic artery occlusion.
- Anterior ischemic optic neuropathy (AION).
- *Retinal vein occlusion (RVO).*

13.2.1.5 Treatment/Management

Thus far, there is no gold standard treatment for CRAO. All proposed therapies are aimed at restoring retinal perfusion. Clinical management currently includes conservative treatments such as a. immediate digital ocular massage to induce oscillations of intraocular pressure and dislodge the offending thrombus; b. topical IOP-lowering therapies with *acetazolamide*, *mannitol*, topical *timolol*, or anterior chamber paracentesis; c. hyperventilation into a paper bag or inhaled 10% carbon dioxide to induce respiratory acidosis and vasodilation. Relatively aggressive treatments are also available, including *thrombolysis* by administering a thrombolytic agent, isovolumic hemodilution, hyperbaric oxygen, reduction of red blood cell rigidity by giving pentoxifylline, systemic steroids intravenously to reduce vascular *endothelial* edema following CRAO, neodymium: yttrium aluminum garnet(YAG) laser arteriotomy and *embolectomy*, cannulation of the supraorbital artery and retrograde injection of antispasmodic papaverine, direct massage of the CRA, and glutamate receptor antagonists.

13.2.2 Retinal Vein Occlusion(RVO)

Retinal vein occlusion(RVO) is the second most common retinal vascular disease *after diabetic retinopathy*. It can be divided into the following two types according to the location of the obstruction: central retinal vein occlusion (CRVO) and branch retinal vein occlusion

(BRVO). Of the two main types of RVO, branch retinal vein occlusion (BRVO) is more prevalent than central retinal vein occlusion (CRVO).

Central retinal vein occlusion(CRVO) remains a common cause of unilateral visual loss. CRVO has been traditionally classified into ischemic and non-ischemic based on the degree of capillary non-perfusion on fluorescein angiography. Differentiating both subtypes is important because it allows us to predict the natural history of these patients and how they will respond to therapy. Non-ischemic CRVO is the most common, accounting for about 70% of cases. Ischemic CRVO can be the primary or progression of a non-ischemic CRVO, although progression is not common. The ischemic subtype of CRVO accounts for about 30% of cases and is associated with worse initial presenting visual acuity (VA) and poor visual prognosis even after edema resolution.

A further type called hemi-vein occlusion was previously diagnosed as BRVO. In most of the current studies, hemi-CRVO is defined as a particular form of CRVO. BRVO is divided, depending on which venous branch is affected, into two forms: major BRVO and macular BRVO.

13.2.2.1 Risk factors

CRVO presents mainly in older individuals, with over 90% of cases occurring in persons older than 50. An increased risk of CRVO has been shown in patients with *systemic arteriosclerotic vascular disease*, hypertension, *diabetes mellitus, dyslipidemia*, high body mass index, smoking, and glaucoma. Other risk factors are different forms of vasculitis, neoplasia, and drugs such as oral contraceptives or diuretics.

BRVO refers to the obstruction of a branch of the retinal vein at an *arteriovenous* crossing. This compression of the vein is thought to cause turbulent blood flow that leads to thrombus formation. It can have multiple underlying causes, including age, hypertension, diabetic retinopathy, or hypercoagulability.

13.2.2.2 Pathogenesis

The exact pathogenesis of RVO remains unclear. The condition may be due to a combination of three systemic changes known as Virchow's triad: venous stasis, endothelial damage, and hypercoagulability. Any cause of reduced venous outflow, damage to the venous vasculature, or hypercoagulable states places the patient at an increased risk for central retinal vein occlusion. Hyperopia and glaucoma have been reported as local ophthalmic risk factors. The increased intraocular pressure in glaucoma can compromise retinal vein outflow and produce stasis.

13.2.2.3 Symptoms and clinical features

Patients with CRVO usually present with sudden, painless, unilateral loss of vision. However, patients with BRVO can be *asymptomatic*, or they may present with blurred vision, usually involving the sector of the visual field corresponding to the area of the occluded venous branch. Generally, macular edema is the most important cause of reduced vision in patients with RVO.

Characteristic clinical features are flame-shaped, dot or blot retinal hemorrhages, and dilated tortuous veins with optic disc oedema, cotton wool spots, and cystoid macular oedema. In CRVO the retinal hemorrhages and *exudates* are distributed throughout all four quadrants. BRVO occurs more frequently in the *superotemporal* and *inferotemporal* quadrants.

Common ocular investigations for RVO include *fluorescein angiography (FA)* and optical coherence tomography (OCT). There is usually a variable delay in retinal vascular filling because of the obstruction to venous outflow in a vascular system. The later phases of the angiogram will show variable staining of the optic nerve head and retinal veins together with variable degrees of vascular leakage in the macular and capillary nonperfusion. OCT will often show cystic fluid-filled spaces in the macular with retinal thickening and occasionally submacular fluid. Currently, the exact measurement of macular edema is available using OCT. The latest generation of spectral-domain OCT enables a very accurate measurement of retinal volume in the macular region and exact remeasurement of the same area in follow-up visits.

13.2.2.4 Differential diagnosis

In the differential diagnosis, ocular ischemic syndrome, diabetic and radiation retinopathy, and venous occlusion due to systemic vasculitis have to be excluded.

13.2.2.5 Complications

Complications of this include macular edema, vitreous hemorrhage, traction retinal detachment and neovascular glaucoma.

13.2.2.6 Treatment/Management

Current treatments focus on the *sequelae* of RVO, such as macular edema and retinal *neovascularization*.

The two general approaches to treating RVO are pharmacologic management and surgical intervention. Pharmacologic management of RVO involves *intravitreal* injections of anti-VEGF therapy and/or corticosteroids. In patients with central retinal vein occlusion, vascular endothelial growth factor (VEGF) is elevated; this leads to swelling as well as neovascularization that is prone to bleeding. Intravitreal injections of an anti-VEGF drug to reduce the new blood vessel growth and swelling. Intravitreal corticosteroid injections can have unwanted side effects of cataract formation and intraocular pressure elevations.

Surgical interventions include laser photocoagulation, optic nerve sheath decompression, radial optic neurotomy and *vitrectomy*.

Retinal photocoagulation can be done to treat neovascularization, with the goal of devitalizing some of the retinal tissue to prevent further neovascularization and treat iris neovascularization.

Optic nerve sheath decompression: Sectioning of the posterial scleral ring via an orbital approach is associated with a significant risk, and it is now no longer practiced.

Radical optic neurotomy: The theoretical basis of radial optic neurotomy (RON) remains contentious.

Pars plana vitrectomy (PPV) can be done when central retinal vein occlusions have an associated vitreous hemorrhage.

13.2.2.7 Prognosis

Central retinal vein occlusion has a better prognosis in younger patients. One-third of older patients improve without treatment, one-third stay the same, and one-third get worse. If the central retinal vein occlusion does not become ischemic, return to baseline or near baseline vision occurs in about 50% of patients. In most cases, the prognosis correlates with initial visual acuity. Chronic macular edema is the main cause of poor vision. Ischemic central retinal vein occlusion has a more variable prognosis due to macular ischemia. Patients have a high risk of neovascular glaucoma.

Branch retinal vein occlusion typically has a good prognosis, one important prognostic factor for final visual acuity(VA) appears to be the initial VA.

13.3 MACULOPATHY

13.3.1 Age-Related Macular Degeneration (AMD)

Age-related macular degeneration (AMD) affects one in eight people 60 years of age or older and is the most common cause of irreversible blindness in older persons in developed countries. According to thorough estimates, AMD is estimated to be present in 8.69% of the global population, affecting 196 million people in 2020; this prevalence is expected to increase to 288 million by 2040. The demographic shift brought on by an aging global population can be used to explain the expected increase in the prevalence of adults suffering from non-communicable eye disorders such as AMD. Due to its chronic character, which necessitates consistent long-term management, AMD has become and will remain a public health concern for both high- and low-income countries, with significant socioeconomic ramifications and increases in healthcare costs. Although AMD remains the third leading cause of severe irreversible vision loss worldwide, legal blindness and visual impairment have decreased in incidence since the introduction of treatments targeting vascular endothelial growth factor (VEGF).

13.3.1.1 Risk factors

Several risk factors have been identified and associated with this disease. Risk factors can be classified into sociodemographic, lifestyle, cardiovascular, hormonal and reproductive, inflammatory, genetic, and ocular. Sociodemographic factors include age, gender, race, and socioeconomic status.

Aging is a strong risk factor for the development of AMD. The blue iris is more likely to develop AMD than the brown iris. Systemic factors such as cardiovascular disease are also risk factors for AMD. Elevated blood pressure and atherosclerosis can increase the risk of AMD. The presence of diabetic retinopathy (DR), high-density *lipoprotein* (HDL), obesity and high systolic blood pressure increase the risk of AMD in diabetic patients. Smoking is an independent risk factor for AMD. Alcohol intake is associated with the development of AMD. Lutein and zeaxanthin can reduce the risk of AMD, vitamin C, vitamin E, vitamin D, and zinc oxide can prevent the occurrence of AMD. Increasing fish intake can reduce the risk of AMD. DHA, and EPA may slow the occurrence of AMD.

13.3.1.2 Pathogenesis

The exact pathogenesis of age-related macular degeneration remains unclear, but it is likely to be the result of multifactorial processes. The complicated etiology of AMD has been connected to cellular, biochemical, and molecular processes and is impacted by a number of variables, including both environmental influences and *genetic predisposition*, despite the fact that the pathogenesis of AMD is presently not fully known. Several pathogenic mechanisms can cause AMD at the molecular and biochemical levels. These consist of oxidative damage, aberrant lipid metabolism, apoptosis, structural changes to outer photoreceptor segments, RPE ion channel malfunction, immune system changes, and abnormalities of the extracellular matrix. There are differences in the extracellular matrix composition across the retina, and any modification, such as depletion, synthesis, or enhanced breakdown and waste, can result in retinal alterations linked to AMD.

13.3.1.3 Symptoms and clinical features

Age-related macular degeneration has been classified into two clinical forms dry or non-neovascular and wet or neovascular.

Vision loss is gradual if it occurs in the early or intermediate dry stage of AMD. The examination of the fundus reveals yellowish subretinal deposits or *drusen* and RPE hyperpigmentation or hypopigmentary changes. Drusen can be hard or soft, or they may confluence into larger drusen and may evolve into drusenoid RPE detachments (PED). Atrophy of the *retinal pigment epithelium* occurs in the advanced stage of the disease known as Geographic atrophy. Geographic atrophy involving the center of the macula leads to significant visual loss. Patients with wet AMD typically report visual distortion or blurring of central vision, especially their near vision. Other patients report *metamorphopsia*, *micropsia*, or *scotoma*.

1) Epidemiological classification
- Early AMD: Large (≥125 μm) drusen or retinal pseudodrusen, or pigmentary abnormalities.
- Late AMD: Neovascular AMD or geographic atrophy.

2) Basic clinical classification
- No aging changes: No drusen and no pigment abnormalities.
- Normal aging changes: Only small drusen ≤63 μm and no pigment abnormalities.
- Early AMD: Medium drusen >63 μm and ≤125 μm, and no pigment abnormalities.
- Intermediate AMD: Large drusen >125 μm or any pigment abnormalities.
- Late AMD: Neovascular AMD or geographic atrophy.

3) AREDS simplified severity scale points

0 No large drusen (>125 μm) or pigment changes in either eye.

1 Large drusen or pigment changes in one eye only.

2 Large drusen and pigment changes in one eye only; or large drusen or pigment changes in both eyes; or neovascular AMD or geographic atrophy in one eye.

3 Large drusen and pigment changes in one eye; and large drusen or pigment changes in the fellow eye.

4 Large drusen and pigment changes in both eyes.

13.3.1.4 Differential diagnosis

Differential diagnosis of age-related macular degeneration depends on the stage of the disease. Drusen are also present in the complement component 3 glomerulopathies. Retinal flecks, such as those seen in Stargardt's disease, can be misinterpreted as age-related macular degeneration. The differential diagnosis for CNV from wet AMD should include other causes of CNV.

13.3.1.5 Treatment/Management

1) Treatment of wet AMD

Anti-VEGF agents: Effective treatment for neovascular AMD is based on inhibition of the angiogenic protein VEGF, which is produced in the retina and induced by hypoxia and other conditions. VEGF increases retinal vascular permeability and promotes neovascularisation.

2) Treatment of dry AMD

Progressive dry AMD has no proven effective treatment, unlike wet AMD. Complement inhibition has been identified as an important potential therapeutic intervention for atrophic AMD. However, stem cell-based treatments, a component of regenerative medicine, have produced encouraging outcomes for degenerative retinal conditions such as AMD.

13.3.1.6 Prognosis

Over 2~3 years without treatment, 50%~60% of eyes with wet AMD and subfoveal CNV will lose 6 or more lines of vision, compared to 20%~30% of eyes with any submacular CNV. Classic CNV is associated with worse visual outcomes than occult or minimally classic CNV, and up to half of the patients with no classic lesions on initial presentation may develop classic CNV within a year after diagnosis.

13.3.2 Central Serous Chorioretinopathy(CSC)

Central serous chorioretinopathy (CSC) is a common ocular disease characterized by serous retinal detachment most commonly at the macula, usually associated with pigment epithelial detachments (PED), retinal pigment epithelial (RPE) dysfunction, and choroidal thickening, hyperpermeability, and venous overload. Typical presentations include loss of central vision, central scotoma, micropsia, or metamorphopsia. It is usually unilateral and predominantly affects young or middle-aged adults, with men being affected more frequently than women.

13.3.2.1 Risk factors

- Corticosteroids: Exogenous corticosteroid usage is the most recognized risk factor for CSC.
- Aldosterone and testosterone: Primary hyperaldosteronism has also been associated with CSC. The predominance of CSC in working-aged males has led to the theory that higher levels of androgens such as testosterone may be associated with its pathogenesis.
- Pregnancy: Pregnancy is associated with CSC, potentially due to elevated levels of endogenous corticosteroid, changes in testosterone, the renin-angiotensin system and blood volume, psychological stress, systemic hypertension, and/or pre-eclampsia.
- Systemic hypertension.
- Organ transplantation.
- Psychological stress.
- Sleep disturbance and obstructive sleep apnoea: Poor sleep quality and sleep disturbance have been associated with CSC.
- Genetics and family history.
- Phosphodiesterase-6 inhibitors.
- Hyperopia: Hyperopia is significantly associated with an increased risk of CSC.
- Helicobacter pylori.
- Smoking.
- Alcohol.

13.3.2.2 Pathogenesis

The understanding of the pathophysiology of CSC remains incomplete. Roughly including the following three mechanisms: venous overload choroidopathy and increased scleral thickness; RPE dysfunction; and the role of corticosteroids.

CSC may appear in 2 basic forms: acute and chronic. The acute episode generally resolves within 3 to 6 months. If fluid persists beyond this period, it is called "chronic CSC".

13.3.2.3 Symptoms and clinical features

Acute CSC typically presents with unilateral blurred vision, central scotoma, metamorphopsia, *dyschromatopsia*, micropsia, hypermetropisation, and reduced contrast sensitivity. As the disease has a predilection for the macula, symptoms are usually confined to the central visual field.

On biomicroscopy, there is a well-defined circular or oval area of neurosensory detachment over the posterior pole. The subretinal fluid (SRF) in CSC is commonly clear. However, deposits (with a fibrinous appearance on OCT) may be present in the subretinal space. Abnormalities of the RPE are often present including PED, with RPE atrophy and hyper- and hypo-pigmentation becoming increasingly common as the disease progresses towards chronic CSC. Atypical CSC can present as large bullous serous retinal detachments that are often associated with RPE tears.

13.3.2.4 Differential diagnosis

The differential diagnosis of serous *maculopathy* includes a broad range of diseases. Include ocular neovascular diseases, vitelliform lesions, inflammatory diseases, ocular tumors, hematological malignancies, paraneoplastic syndromes, inherited retinal dystrophies, ocular development anomalies, medication-related conditions and toxicity-related disease, *rhegmatogenous* retinal detachment, and tractional retinal detachment, retinal vascular disease, as well as a miscellaneous category that includes serous maculopathy secondary to RPE dysfunction due to confluent drusen, serous maculopathy with absence of RPE, and serous maculopathy due to aspecific choroidopathy.

Distinguishing between these diseases requires multimodal imaging, often including OCT, OCT-A, FA, FAF, and/or ICGA. In addition to the clinical characteristics such as male preponderance and age at onset of 20~55 years, several key findings on imaging help differentiate between CSC and other diseases. These findings include one or more PEDs on OCT; increased choroidal thickness with dilated vessels in Haller's layer (pachyvessels) often associated with a thinned overlying choriocapillaris and RPE changes; focal or multifocal leakage on FA; and perhaps one of the most typical signs of CSC or pachychoroid disease spectrum, one or more areas of indistinct hyperfluorescence in the affected eye and often the fellow eye as well on mid-phase ICGA.

13.3.2.5 Treatment/Management

In all patients with CSC, avoidance of modifiable risk factors should first be emphasized, both at the time of presentation and lifelong. Most commonly, this involves cessation or avoidance of corticosteroids.

The prognosis for resolution and visual recovery in patients with acute CSC is usually good, thus observation and patient reassurance are considered the best treatment course. Most affected patients recover spontaneously with improvement of visual acuity, reattachment of the sensory retina, and improvement of the other symptoms within 3~4 months. Treatment should be considered in patients with persistent or recurrent SRF to minimize the risk of permanent visual impairment.

Treatment modalities can be classified into laser, systemic medications, intravitreal therapy, and surgery. Of these, faster regression of subretinal exudation may be obtained using laser photocoagulation applied to close focal sites of RPE leakage, or by *photodynamic therapy (PDT)* applied to the areas of choroidal vascular hyperpermeability.

13.3.2.6 Prognosis

In most cases of acute forms of CSC, spontaneous resorption of SRF takes place within 3 months of the onset of the pathology, with adjustment of visual functions with final central VA often of 0.8 and better. However, even despite the improvement of central VA, after the subsidence of the disease patients may complain of dyschromatopsia, reduced contrast sensitivity, metamorphopsia, central scotoma, and in rare cases night blindness.

13.4 RETINITIS PIGMENTOSA (RP)

Retinitis pigmentosa (RP) is an inherited retinal *neurodegenerative* disease characterized by progressive photoreceptor cell death and retinal pigmented epithelium (RPE) atrophy, which initially manifests as *nyctalopia*, followed by continuous vision loss until blindness. It is also called rod-cone dystrophy, due to the primary degeneration of rods rather than cones.

13.4.1 Pathogenesis

The majority of patients have symptoms of diminished peripheral vision on both an upper and lower visual field, as well as night vision loss. Night blindness and peripheral vision are caused by rod cell degeneration. AD-inherited RP is caused by mutations in pre-mRNA splicing. The X-linked RP is caused by mutations in the RPGR and RP2 genes at their respective loci. Multiple mutations result in photoreceptor cells degenerating.

The fundus examination reveals the loss in retinal blood vessels in addition to the peripheral bone-spicule deposits. ERG is the prosperous diagnostic standard, showing the reduction in the rod and the cone response that are united with a delay in their timing. The visual field (VF) loss is a crucial indicator since it shows the disease's course and the effectiveness of treatment, ranging from patchy loss of the peripheral visual region to tunnel vision, ring scotoma, and eventually leading to total blindness.

13.4.2 Symptoms and Clinical Features

Night blindness. The initial symptom of RP is usually defective dark adaptation. Usually, this includes a relatively vague sense of being unable to see well in low-light situations or those requiring rapid adaptation from light to dim environments. Narrowing of the visual fields is not initially obvious but will become apparent over time.

Visual acuity. Central visual acuity is usually preserved until the end stages of RP. Central acuity loss can occur at all ages from cystoid macular edema (CME), which is estimated to occur in approximately 10%~50% of individuals with RP.

Fundus appearance includes the "classic triad" seen on a fundoscopic exam of bony spicule pigmentation, vascular narrowing, and abnormal pallor of the optic disc. These may not be evident early in the disease, and the degree to which abnormalities are seen is variable with the severity of the disease. Other associated physical findings may include subcapsular cataracts and macular edema.

13.4.3 Differential Diagnosis

The list of differential diagnoses in RP is extensive and includes infectious (e.g., syphilis or congenital rubella), drug-induced (e.g., chloroquine or thioridazine), iatrogenic (e.g., laser photocoagulation), metabolic (e.g., gyrate atrophy due to hyperornithinemia) and nutritional etiologies (e.g., vitamin A and zinc deficiencies), as well as a range of non-RP-inherited retinal dystrophies (e.g., choroideremia, congenital stationary night blindness and Oguchi disease). In addition, it is important to rule out several metabolic diseases that may present with fundus findings mimicking RP, including abetalipoproteinemia (Bassen-Kornzweig disease), ataxia with vitamin E deficiency, and adult Refsum disease, among others.

13.4.4 Treatment/Management

There is presently no cure or effective medication available to delay or stop the progression of the condition. Most of the pharmacological therapies discovered nowadays try to improve patients' quality of life. Some curative therapies, with the ability to slow down photoreceptors' degeneration and preserve healthy ones, have been developed.

13.4.4.1 Antioxidant agents

The principal function of these agents is to prevent photoreceptors' death and so preserve the visual acuity.

13.4.4.2 Hyperbaric oxygen

Hyperbaric oxygen (HBO) therapy exposes the patient to a barometric pressure higher than the sea level ambient pressure, increasing the transfer of oxygen into tissues.

13.4.4.3 Stem cell therapy

The purpose of this type of therapy is to introduce stem cells, which can differentiate into retinal cells. Cell-based therapy works to replace retinal tissue with effective stem cells, restore dysfunctional cells by releasing trophic factors, and create new synapses.

13.4.4.4 Gene therapy

With gene therapy, by using different types of vectors, it is possible to bring a wild-type gene into the affected cells, promoting the expression of the working protein and suppressing the mutated one.

13.4.5 Prognosis

The prognosis for patients with retinitis pigmentosa is dependent on the age of onset and pattern of inheritance. Early-onset symptoms such as severe vision loss and night blindness are expected with the autosomal recessive form of RP. The autosomal dominant expression is the least severe and is associated with the more gradual onset of symptoms later in adult life. The most severe vision loss occurs with X-linked recessive RP. Tunnel vision is expected late in the course of all forms of RP, and almost all RP patients will be legally blind at some point in the progression of their disease. Total loss of vision is fortunately uncommon, as the macular function will generally allow light perception, even after acuity is lost.

13.5 SYSTEMIC DISEASES AND RETINOPATHY

13.5.1 Hypertensive Retinopathy

Hypertension affects the eyes through a series of pathophysiological modifications that can damage the retinal, choroidal, and optic nerve circulations causing respectively retinopathy, choroidopathy, and optic neuropathy. Hypertensive retinopathy (HR) occurs when the retinal vessels get damaged due to elevated blood pressure.

13.5.1.1 Pathogenesis

Retinal *microvascular* signs of HR may be caused by an acute increase in systemic blood pressure or by chronic elevated hypertension. HR has been associated with endothelial cell dysfunction, low-grade systemic inflammation, and oxidative stress. The pathophysiology of HR can be divided into three phases of histologic damage.

In the first phase or "vasoconstrictive phase", the initial response to elevated blood pressure is constituted by localized vasospasm and vasoconstriction of the retinal arterioles.

Elevated blood pressure over time leads to structural changes in the vessel wall such as endothelial damage, intimal thickening, media-wall hyperplasia, and hyaline degeneration. This phase is called the "sclerotic phase", which results in arteriovenous crossing change or nicking, and accentuation of focal or diffuse light reflex of vessel walls. Arteriovenous nicking occurs when a thickened arteriole crosses the venule where the vessels have their common adventitial sheath.

The "exudative phase" is seen in patients with severe systemic hypertension. This late phase leads to disruption of the blood-retina barrier causing haemorrhages in the superficial or inner retinal layers or exudation of lipids seen as hard exudates. This subsequently causes cotton wool spots.

Finally, very severe and long-standing systemic hypertension can lead to a condition called "malignant hypertension" characterized by elevated intracranial pressure which causes optic nerve ischemia and optic disc swelling.

13.5.1.2 Symptoms and clinical features

Hypertensive retinopathy is usually asymptomatic and is diagnosed on fundoscopic features. The following are signs of hypertensive retinopathy:

- AV crossing changes.
- Arterial changes: Decrease in the arteriovenous ratio to 1:3 (the normal ratio is 2:3).
- Change in the arteriolar light reflex (light reflex appears as copper and/or silver wiring).
- Retinal changes: Retinal hemorrhages and retinal exudates.
- Optic nerve changes: Optic disk swelling (also known as hypertensive optic neuropathy).

Classification based on different clinical signs:

- None: No detectable signs.
- Mild: Generalized arteriolar narrowing, focal arteriolar narrowing, arteriovenous nicking, arteriolar wall opacification (silver or copper wiring), or a combination of these signs.
- Moderate: Hemorrhages (blot, dot, or flame-shaped), microaneurysms, cotton-wool

spots, hard exudates, or a combination of these signs.
- Malignant: Signs of moderate retinopathy in combination with optic disc swelling, in the presence of severely elevated blood pressure.

13.5.1.3 Differential diagnosis

The other conditions that present with optic disc swelling are diabetic papillopathy, central retinal vein occlusion, anterior ischemic optic neuropathy, and neuroretinitis. Conditions that mimic chronic hypertensive retinopathy are diabetic retinopathy, retinal venous obstruction, hyperviscosity syndrome, ocular ischemic syndrome, and radiation retinopathy.

13.5.1.4 Treatment/Management

Before treatment is considered, a thorough history should be obtained. Patients should be asked about the duration, symptoms, and secondary complications (stroke, heart failure, renal failure, and peripheral vascular disease) of hypertension. The treatment of hypertensive retinopathy is primarily focused on reducing systemic blood pressure. If vision-threatening retinal pathology is present, treatment may be warranted. Some studies have reported data regarding the management of acute hypertension retinopathy with intravitreal injections of anti-VEGF agents.

13.5.2 Diabetic Retinopathy (DR)

As the worldwide prevalence of diabetes mellitus continues to increase, diabetic retinopathy remains a leading cause of vision loss in many developed countries. Diabetic retinopathy (DR) is an important microvascular complication. Of the 246 million people with diabetes, about a third have signs of diabetic retinopathy, and a third of these might have vision-threatening retinopathy, defined as severe retinopathy or macular oedema. Apart from its effects on vision, the presence of diabetic retinopathy also signifies a heightened risk of life-threatening systemic vascular complications.

13.5.2.1 Risk factors

The development of diabetic retinopathy strongly correlates with a longer duration of diabetes, greater hyperglycemia, and hypertension. The most important treatable risk factor for the development of DR is hyperglycemia. A higher HbA1c level is significantly associated with the progression of diabetic retinopathy and intensive glycemic control reduces the incidence and deterioration of retinopathy. Moreover, there is clear evidence regarding the relationship between hypertension and diabetic retinopathy. Puberty and pregnancy are well-known risk factors for diabetic retinopathy in people with type 1 diabetes. Diabetic retinopathy is associated with many other systemic and lifestyle factors, including nephropathy, obesity, alcohol consumption, and haematological markers of anaemia, hypothyroidism, inflammation, and endothelial dysfunction.

13.5.2.2 Pathogenesis

Chronic exposure to hyperglycaemia and other causal risk factors (e.g., hypertension) is believed to initiate a cascade of biochemical and physiological changes that ultimately lead to microvascular damage and retinal dysfunction. Various mechanisms account for the features of diabetic retinopathy. Histopathologic analysis shows thickening of capillary basement membranes, microaneurysm formation, loss of pericytes, capillary acellularity, and neovascularization. Microaneurysms, outpouchings of the capillary wall, serve as sites of fluid and lipid leakage, which can lead to the development of diabetic macular edema. Theories on the biochemistry of these end-organ changes include toxic effects from sorbitol accumulation, vascular damage by excessive glycosylation with crosslinking of basement membrane proteins, and activation of protein kinase C-ß2 by vascular endothelial growth factor (VEGF), leading to increased vascular permeability and endothelial cell proliferation. VEGF, produced by the retina in response to hypoxia, is believed to play a central role in the development of neovascularization.

13.5.2.3 Symptoms and clinical features

Patients might be asymptomatic in the early stages and might be discovered incidentally on fundus examination. As the disease progresses, the symptoms include blurred vision, distorted vision, floaters, and partial or total vision loss.

1) Clinical features
- Microaneurysms are the earliest clinically detectable lesions.
- Hemorrhages: Weakened capillary wall ruptures lead to intraretinal dot hemorrhages.
- Hard exudates: They are composed of lipoprotein and lipid-filled macrophages located in the outer plexiform layer.
- Soft exudates: They are located in the retinal nerve fiber layer and represent focal infarcts of the precapillary arterioles.
- Intraretinal microvascular abnormalities (IRMA) : IRMAs are intercommunications between retinal arteriole and venules.
- Venous changes.
- Neovascularization: Neovascularization at the disc (NVD) is defined as neovascularization at or within one disc diameter of the optic disc. Neovascularization elsewhere (NVE) is defined as a new vessel away from one disc diameter of the optic disc. Neovascularization of iris (NVI) is a marker of poor prognosis and is associated with the propensity to develop neovascular glaucoma.

2) Early treatment diabetic retinopathy study (ETDRS) classification
- No retinopathy: No microvascular lesions.
- Mild non-proliferative diabetic retinopathy (NPDR) : Microaneurysms only.
- Moderate NPDR: Microaneurysms and other microvascular lesions, but not severe NPDR.
- Severe NPDR: More than 20 intraretinal haemorrhages in four quadrants venous beading in two or more quadrants, or intraretinal microvascular abnormalities in one or more quadrants but not proliferative diabetic retinopathy.

- *Proliferative diabetic retinopathy*: Neovascularisation of the optic disc (NVD) or elsewhere (NVE), preretinal haemorrhage, or vitreous haemorrhage; high-risk characteristics are mild NVD with vitreous haemorrhage, moderate-to-severe NVD with or without vitreous haemorrhage; moderate NVE with vitreous haemorrhage.
- Clinically significant macular oedema: Retinal thickening within 500 μm from centre of the macula; hard exudates within 500 μm from centre of the macula with adjacent retinal thickening; retinal thickening of more than one optic disc area within one optic disc diameter from centre of the macula.

13.5.2.4 Screening

As diabetic retinopathy remains the leading cause of visual impairment, screening for diabetic retinopathy is important to early detect preventable blindness. Most patients with developed diabetic retinopathy have no symptoms until *macular edema (ME)* or proliferative diabetic retinopathy (PDR) presents. Although *panretinal laser photocoagulation (PRP)* and intraocular VEGF inhibitor injection are effective for ME or PDR related visual impairment, they benefit more in preventing visual loss than in reversing deteriorated visual acuity. Therefore, a timely screening program for diabetic retinopathy could assist individuals with diabetes to preserve their vision.

The American Academy of Ophthalmology has recommended screening for diabetic retinopathy 5 years after diagnosis in patients with type 1 diabetes, and at the time of diagnosis in patients with type 2 diabetes.

13.5.2.5 Differential diagnosis

- Central retinal vein occlusion.
- Hypertensive retinopathy.
- Sickle cell retinopathy.
- Terson syndrome.
- Ocular ischemic syndrome.
- Branch retinal vein occlusion.
- Hemiretinal vein occlusion.
- Valsalva retinopathy.
- Post-traumatic retinal bleed.
- Retinal macroaneurysm.
- Retinopathy in thalassemia.

13.5.2.6 Complications

Vision-threatening complications associated with poorly controlled diabetic retinopathy include diabetic macular edema, tractional retinal detachment, and vitreous hemorrhage as a late sequela of proliferative diabetic retinopathy.

13.5.2.7 Treatment/Management

In addition to optimal medical control of blood glucose, blood pressure, and serum cholesterol level, several intraocular managements have become standard treatments for diabetic retinopathy. As for patients with diabetic macular edema (DME), the use of anti-VEGF therapy has reformed its management.

For patients with proliferative diabetic retinopathy, panretinal laser photocoagulation has been demonstrated to be effective in reducing the risk of vision loss. PRP, therefore, is considered the preferred treatment for patients with all stages of PDR and severe NPDR. In addition to PRP, recent studies have also provided evidence that intravitreous injection of anti-VEGF may be a safe alternative treatment for PDR.

Vitrectomy has been the mainstay surgical treatment for the two blinding complications of advanced retinopathy—persistent vitreous haemorrhage and tractional retinal detachment.

13.6 RETINAL DETACHMENT (RD)

Retinal detachment (RD) occurs when the neurosensory retina, the neurovascular tissue responsible for phototransduction, is separated from the underlying retinal pigment epithelium (RPE). There are three main types of RD: rhegmatogenous, tractional, and exudative RD. In rhegmatogenous RD, one or more retinal breaks enable vitreous fluid to enter the subretinal space and separate the neurosensory retina from the RPE. In tractional RD, preretinal, intraretinal, or subretinal membranes contract and exert tangential forces and elevate the retina from the underlying RPE. Finally, in exudative RD, an underlying inflammatory condition, vascular abnormality or the presence of a tumour causes exudative fluid to accumulate in the subretinal space, exceeding the osmotic pump function of the RPE.

13.6.1 Risk Factors

Rhegmatogenous retinal detachment(RRD): Elderly, highly myopic, aphakic, intraocular lens, eye trauma,previous retinal detachment in the other eye.

Tractional retinal detachments(TRD): Proliferative diabetic retinopathy, proliferative vitreoretinopathy, retinal vascular disease complicated with vitreous hemorrhage, retinopathy of prematurity, and trauma.

Exudative retinal detachment(ERD): Primary ocular tumors; ocular metastases; sarcoidosis; syphilis; toxoplasmosis; sympathetic ophthalmia; central serous chorioretinopathy; polypoidal choroidal vasculopathy; tuberculosis; corticosteroid therapy; Vogt-Koyanagi-Harada syndrome; pre-eclampsia, eclampsia; organ transplantation; optic nerve pit; acute retinal necrosis; coats disease.

13.6.2 Pathogenesis

A rhegmatogenous retinal detachment is when a tear, break, or hole occurs in the retina.

Tractional retinal detachments: When there are proliferative membranes in the vitreous or on the retinal surface, these membranes can pull on the neurosensory retina. When the force is strong enough, it can separate the neurosensory retina from the underlying RPE.

Exudative retinal detachments: In these detachments, subretinal fluid accumulates due to fluid exudation from a large lesion, such as a tumor or inflammatory mediators.

13.6.3 Symptoms and Clinical Features

Patients with an RRD may present with a history of a large number of new-onset floaters. They may also have significant photopsia in their vision. The patient often presents with slowly progressive or fixed visual field loss, typically starting in the periphery and then moving centrally.

13.6.4 Treatment/Management

Management of RRD and TRD is typically surgical. ERD usually has nonsurgical management. If the patient has an RRD, the surgeon should identify and seal all retinal breaks or tears. In TRD, tractional elements must be relieved. For ERD, management is nonsurgical. The underlying retinal or choroidal disease or mass should be identified and treated.

13.6.5 Prognosis

The success rate of surgery is over 90%, and the visual prognosis depends on whether the macula is detached and the duration of detachment. The patient may be at higher risk for PVR if they are older, have giant retinal tears, retinal detachments involving more than two quadrants, vitreous hemorrhage, a choroidal detachment, had a previous retinal detachment repair, or if using cryotherapy.

Chapter 14
Strabismus and Nystagmus

INTRODUCTION
- ▶ Strabismus
- ▶ Nystagmus
- ▶ Anatomy and Physiology of the Ocular Motility System

STRABISMUS
- ▶ Esotropia
- ▶ Exotropia

MANAGEMENT OF STRABISMUS
- ▶ Basis for Treatment
- ▶ Available Treatment Options
- ▶ Management Strategies for Strabismus
- ▶ Patient Education

NYSTAGMUS
- ▶ Etiology
- ▶ Features of Nystagmus
- ▶ Types of Nystagmus
- ▶ Nystagmus Movements
- ▶ Management for Nystagmus

14.1 INTRODUCTION

14.1.1 Strabismus

The tendency for the eyes to deviate from each other can be classified as "*latent*" when the eyes are kept in alignment by the fusion mechanism and "*manifest*" when alignment is not maintained by fusion. Latent deviation of the eyes is called *heterophoria*; manifest deviation is called *heterotropia* or *strabismus*.

14.1.2 Nystagmus

It is defined as regular and rhythmic to-and-fro involuntary *oscillatory* movements of the eyes.

14.1.3 Anatomy and Physiology of the Ocular Motility System

14.1.3.1 Extraocular muscles

A set of six extraocular muscles (4 recti and 2 obliques) control the movements of each eye. *Rectus muscles* are superior (SR), inferior (IR), medial (MR) and lateral (LR). The *oblique muscles* include superior (SO) and inferior (IO). The primary and secondary functions of each extraocular muscle are shown in *Table 14-1*.

Table 14-1 The actions of extraocular muscles

Muscle	Primary action	Secondary action	Tertiary action
MR	Adduction	-	-
LR	Abduction	-	-
SR	Elevation	Intorsion	Adduction
IR	Depression	Extorsion	Adduction
SO	Intorsion	Depression	Abduction
IO	Extorsion	Elevation	Abduction

14.1.3.2 Nerve supply

The extraocular muscles are supplied by third, fourth and sixth cranial nerves. The third *cranial* nerve (*oculomotor*) supplies the superior, medial and inferior recti and inferior oblique muscles. The fourth cranial nerve (*trochlear*) supplies the superior oblique and the sixth nerve (*abducent*) supplies the lateral rectus muscle.

14.1.3.3 Synergists, antagonists and yoke muscles

Synergists: It refers to the muscles having the same primary action in the same eye. For example, superior rectus and inferior oblique of the same eye act as synergistic elevators.

Antagonists: These are the muscles having opposite actions in the same eye. For example, medial and lateral recti, superior and inferior recti and superior and inferior obliques are antagonists to each other in the same eye.

Yoke muscles (contralateral synergists): It refers to the pair of muscles (one from each eye) which contract simultaneously during version movements. For example, right lateral rectus and left medial rectus act as yoke muscles for *dextroversion* movements. Other pairs of yoke muscles are right MR and left LR, right LR and left MR, right SR and left IO, right IR and left SO, right SO and left IR, and right IO and left SR.

Contralateral antagonists: These are a pair of muscles (one from each eye) having opposite action, e.g., right LR and left LR, right MR and left MR.

14.1.3.4 Diagnostic positions of gaze

There are nine diagnostic positions of gaze, including one primary, four secondary and four *tertiary* positions.

Primary position of gaze is the position assumed by the eyes when fixating a distant object (straight ahead) with the erect position of head.

Secondary positions of gaze are the positions assumed by the eyes while looking straight up, straight down, to the right and to the left.

Tertiary positions of gaze describe the positions assumed by the eyes when combination of vertical and horizontal movements occur. These include position of eyes in *dextroelevation*, *dextrodepression*, *levoelevation* and *levodepression*.

Cardinal positions of gaze are the positions which allow examination of each of the 12 extraocular muscles in their main field of action. There are six cardinal positions of gaze, viz, dextroversion, *levoversion*, dextroelevation, levoelevation, dextrodepression and levodepression.

14.2 STRABISMUS

14.2.1 Esotropia

A convergent strabismus is termed an esotropia. Most patients with esotropia present before school age, generally between the ages of 2 and 3 years. Esotropia is often *constant*. In most cases, intermittent esotropia occurs initially in association with accommodative esotropia or *decompensated* esophoria (a tendency of one eye to deviate inward). The intermittency of accommodative esotropia is attributed to the *fluctuating* accommodative status of the patient at the onset of the deviation. Without treatment, intermittent esotropia is likely to become constant. The clinical forms of esotropia are discussed below.

14.2.1.1 Infantile esotropia

When esotropia begins in the developmentally and neurologically normal child during the first 6 months of life, it is classified as "*infantile*". When it occurs after 6 months of age, it is referred to as "early-*acquired*". True "*congenital*" esotropia, which is present at birth, is considered extremely rare; however, the terms "infantile esotropia", "essential infantile esotropia", and "congenital esotropia" are often used interchangeably. The probable age of onset for infantile esotropia is at 2~4 months of age.

14.2.1.2 Acquired esotropia

Acquired forms of esotropia occur at a later age than infantile esotropia. Usually, normal binocular vision has existed prior to the onset of the condition.

1) Accommodative esotropia

This acquired strabismus is associated with the activation of accommodation. The esotropia is attributed partly or totally to either uncorrected hyperopic refractive error and/or a high accommodative convergence/accommodation (AC/A) ratio. Accommodative esotropia has a better understood mechanism and a more straightforward treatment or management than any other form of strabismus. It is reduced partly or entirely by correcting the hyperopic refractive error and/or prescribing a near addition.

2) Nonaccommodative esotropia

An acquired strabismus that develops after 6 months of age, nonaccommodative esotropia is not associated with accommodative effort. Correcting any *coexisting* hyperopia and/or prescribing a near addition for children with nonaccommodative esotropia has minimal or no effect on the size of the esotropia.

3) Acute esotropia

When a convergent strabismus develops suddenly without any apparent *etiology* in a school-aged or older patient with previously normal binocular vision, it is called *acute* esotropia. The sudden diplopia that usually occurs in acute esotropia may result from an underlying and potentially life-threatening disease process, thus it requires immediate evaluation. Its onset can often be traced to a precise hour of a particular day.

4) Mechanical esotropia

A convergent strabismus caused by a mechanical restriction or tightness of an extraocular muscle (e.g., *fibrosis* of muscle tissue, *thyroid myopathy*) or a physical obstruction (e.g., *blowout fracture*) of the extraocular muscles, is classified as a mechanical esotropia. Some patients with Duane syndrome have tightening of the medial and/or lateral recti muscles secondary to the primary underlying neurological miswiring and co-innervation. There is a limitation or absence of abduction, causing an increasing esotropia. The palpebral fissure narrows when the eye rotates inward (adduction). In addition, the patient may exhibit an upshoot or downshoot when the eye *adducts*.

14.2.1.3 Secondary esotropia

An esotropia that results from a *primary* sensory deficit or as a result of surgical intervention is classified as a *secondary* esotropia.

1) Sensory esotropia

A convergent strabismus resulting from *visual deprivation* or *trauma* in one eye that limits *sensory fusion* is classified as a sensory esotropia. It may result from any number of conditions that limit visual acuity in one eye (e.g., uncorrected anisometropia, *unilateral* cataract, corneal *opacity*, optic *atrophy*, and macular disease). It occurs most frequently in persons under 5 years of age. Approximately 4% of those with esotropia have sensory esotropia.

2) Consecutive esotropia

A convergent strabismus that occurs after surgical overcorrection of an exotropia, consecutive esotropia is frequently associated with other oculomotor anomalies (e.g., vertical or *cyclotorsional deviations*). It may result in amblyopia and loss of normal binocular vision in young children and diplopia in adults.

14.2.1.4 Microesotropia

When the angle of esotropia is less than 10 PD, it is classified as microesotropia. This condition often occurs beginning in a child under 3 years of age, and, in some cases, may escape diagnosis by conventional methods. The esotropia is constant and usually unilateral. The terms "microtropia", "microsquint", "minitropia", "monofixation syndrome", and "small-angle deviation" have been used to describe microesotropia.

14.2.2 Exotropia

Exotropia, or divergent strabismus, can be subclassified on the basis of its comparative magnitude at distance and near or its frequency. In basic-type exotropia, the angle of deviation is within 10 PD at distance and near. In the convergence-insufficiency type, the angle of deviation at near exceeds the angle of deviation at distance by at least 10 PD. Divergence-excess type exotropia occurs when the angle of deviation at distance exceeds the angle of deviation at near by at least 10 PD. Although exotropias may be constant or intermittent, most are intermittent. Children with intermittent exotropia often have the divergence-excess type. Other clinical classifications of exotropia are discussed in the following paragraphs.

14.2.2.1 Infantile exotropia

A divergent strabismus that begins during the first 6 months of life is classified as infantile exotropia. It is less common than infantile esotropia. In infants, some cases of constant exotropia may be associated with *neurological* syndromes or defects, *craniofacial* syndromes, and structural abnormalities in the eye.

14.2.2.2 Acquired exotropia

An exotropia occurring after 6 months of age is considered to be acquired rather than infantile.

1) Intermittent exotropia

In intermittent exotropia, the patient sometimes manifests diplopia, *suppression*, or anomalous *retinal correspondence,* and at other times, normal binocular alignment with good stereopsis. The period of strabismus and level of control are variable for each patient. Basic intermittent exotropia accounts for approximately 50% of all cases of intermittent exotropia, with convergence insufficiency and divergence excess making up the balance of cases in approximately equal proportions. Intermittent exotropia typically presents between the ages of 1 and 4 years. In the United States, it occurs in approximately 1% of children by the age of 7 years. Without treatment over the years, intermittent exotropia may either progress (both in degree and the amount of time it is manifest), stay the same, or, in some cases, improve. It rarely *deteriorates* to constant exotropia and fusion and some fixation at distance is usually maintained.

2) Acute exotropia

When a divergent strabismus develops suddenly in an older patient who previously had normal binocular vision, it is classified as acute exotropia. This condition can result from an underlying disease process or a decompensating exophoria.

3) Mechanical exotropia

Mechanical exotropia is a divergent strabismus caused by a mechanical restriction or tightness (e.g., fibrosis of muscle tissue, thyroid myopathy) or a physical obstruction of the extraocular muscles (orbital fracture), causing increasing exotropia. Tightness of the lateral rectus muscle may develop secondary to the primary innervational miswiring in a rare type of Duane syndrome. With this type of strabismus, an absence of adduction results in increasing exotropia accompanied by narrowing of the palpebral fissure and retraction of the globe.

14.2.2.3 Secondary exotropia

An exotropia that results from a primary sensory deficit or occurs as a result of some form of treatment for an esotropia is referred to as a secondary exotropia.

1) Sensory exotropia

A divergent strabismus results from a unilateral decrease in vision that disrupts fusion. Sensory exotropia may be due to a sensory deficit such as uncorrected anisometropia, unilateral cataract, or other unilateral visual impairment.

Sensory exotropia and sensory esotropia occur with equal frequency in children under age 5. However, sensory exotropia predominates in persons older than 5 years. Sensory exotropia occurs in less than 3% of all strabismic children.

2) Consecutive exotropia

Exotropia that occurs following surgical or optical correction of an esotropia is referred to as consecutive exotropia. This form of exotropia can also occur *spontaneously* in a formerly esotropic patient. A spontaneous change from esotropia to exotropia over time may be related to amblyopia of the deviating eye, weak binocular function, underaction of the medial rectus, or excessive hyperopic refractive error. When followed long term, the prevalence of consecutive exotropia is reported to be as high as 20% for esotropic patients treated with surgery.

14.2.2.4 Microexotropia

For a constant exotropia of less than 10 PD, microexotropia occurs much less frequently than microesotropia.

14.3 MANAGEMENT OF STRABISMUS

Management of the strabismic patient is based on the interpretation and analysis of the examination results and overall evaluation. The goals of treatment and management may include:

- Obtaining normal visual acuity in each eye.
- Obtaining and/or improving fusion.
- Eliminating any associated sensory adaptations.
- Obtaining a favorable functional appearance of the alignment of the eyes.

The significance of normal ocular alignment for the development of a positive self-image and interpersonal eye contact cannot be overemphasized.

14.3.1 Basis for Treatment

The indications for treatment and management and the specific types of treatment and management need to be individualized for each patient. In determining a course of therapy, the optometrist should consider the following:

- Age of the patient at the onset of strabismus.
- Current age of the patient.
- Overall health status of the patient.
- Patient's developmental level and anticipated *compliance* with therapy.
- Concerns of the patient and/or parents.
- Symptoms and signs of visual discomfort.
- Visual demands of the patient.
- Comitancy of the deviation.
- Size and frequency of the strabismus.
- Presence or absence of fusion.
- Presence or absence of amblyopia.

14.3.2 Available Treatment Options

The treatment and management of strabismus may include any or all of the following procedures.

14.3.2.1 Optical correction

Regardless of the cause of the strabismus, the goal for strabismic patients, especially very young patients, is to allow binocularity to develop. The best optical correction that allows equally clear retinal images to be formed in each eye is generally the starting point for all treatment and management. However, overcorrection or undercorrection of the refractive error may be prescribed in some instances to affect the angle of strabismus. Hyperopia may be either partly or totally causative in as many as 50% of all cases of esotropia. Anisometropia and astigmatism should also be fully corrected. Whereas a full correction of refractive error is often prescribed for esotropia and hyperopia, the presence of exotropia and hyperopia may require a more *conservative approach*.

14.3.2.2 Added lens power

Lenses can also be used to take advantage of the AC/A ratio to help obtain or maintain binocular vision. A bifocal lens prescription may be used for the patient with fusion potential or when full plus acceptance at distance cannot be attained initially. *Periodic follow-up* is required to determine the efficacy of this treatment and management. Bifocals are often prescribed for the patient with esotropia who has a high AC/A ratio, to eliminate or decrease the angle of strabismus at near to an amount controllable by compensating divergence.

14.3.2.3 Prisms

Ophthalmic prisms can aid in the establishment or maintenance of sensory fusion, by moving the image of the target of regard onto or closer to the fovea of each eye. Prisms are generally prescribed for patients with strabismic deviations of less than 20 PD who are capable of fusion. The presence of amblyopia, deep suppression, and/or anomalous retinal correspondence generally *contraindicates* the use of prisms. *Disruptive* prisms (i.e., overcorrecting or *inverse*) may be prescribed to eliminate anomalous retinal correspondence. In addition, inverse prisms may be used to improve the cosmetic appearance of the strabismic patient who has a poor *prognosis* for attaining normal binocularity and is not interested in surgery.

14.3.2.4 Vision therapy

Vision therapy or orthoptics involves active training procedures to improve the patient's fixation ability and oculomotor control, to help eliminate amblyopia, to improve sensory and *motor fusion*, and to increase facility and the range of accommodation and vergence responses. Used alone or in conjunction with refractive correction, added lens power, prisms, or surgery, these vision therapy procedures are adapted to the individual patient and modified as the patient achieves binocular vision.

14.3.2.5 Extraocular muscle surgery

The clinician should consider all aspects of the nonsurgical treatment of strabismus before recommending surgery. Surgical *consultation* is appropriate for patients whose strabismus is cosmetically objectionable, as well as for patients who may not display the intellectual, motivational, or physiological characteristics (including fusion potential) that warrant consideration of other treatment. In general, surgery for esotropia may be considered when the manifest deviation exceeds 15 PD in the primary position at both distance and near while the patient is wearing the full refractive correction. For patients with exotropia, deviations exceeding 20 PD in the primary position are possible candidates for surgery. Patients with smaller deviations usually should not be considered for surgery, except when adults have acquired symptomatic deviations that do not respond to nonsurgical therapy. Patients with totally accommodative esotropia should not be considered for extraocular muscle surgery, because of the risk of inducing consecutive exotropia.

14.3.2.6 Chemodenervation

The *injection* of *botulinum toxin* type A has been used as either an alternative or an *adjunct* to conventional incisional surgery in selected strabismic patients. The toxin selectively *binds* to *nerve terminals* and interferes with the release of *acetylcholine*, thereby functionally denervating muscles injected with small amounts of the drug. The *dose-related* but temporary *paralysis* of an extraocular muscle leads to a change in eye position, followed by some degree of *contracture* of the opposing muscle.

14.3.3 Management Strategies for Strabismus
14.3.3.1 Accommodative esotropia

After the diagnosis of accommodative esotropia has been confirmed, correction of the amount of hyperopia needed to obtain ocular alignment should be provided. If present, amblyopia should be treated. The clinician may prescribe active vision therapy procedures for the development and enhancement of normal sensory and motor fusion.

14.3.3.2 Acute esotropia and exotropia

Once the cause of the esotropia or exotropia has been determined, prisms may be used to correct small and moderate deviations (except in late-onset accommodative esotropia) to eliminate diplopia and re-establish binocular vision. For larger and *transient* deviations, the optometrist can prescribe *Fresnel prisms*. Vision therapy may be prescribed to expand fusional vergence amplitudes and facility. Surgical consultation may be considered for deviations that have become stable over time, when the angle of deviation exceeds 15~20 PD, and when the strabismus is cosmetically displeasing.

14.3.3.3 Consecutive esotropia and exotropia

Persistent consecutive esotropia following surgery for intermittent exotropia should be treated aggressively in young children, using lenses, prisms, and vision therapy to prevent possible amblyopia and loss of binocular vision. Older patients with consecutive esotropia following surgery frequently have diplopia and usually require similar treatment. Consecutive exotropia that is spontaneous and optically induced can be treated by reducing the power of the hyperopic lenses. This is generally done in younger patients when the exotropia exceeds 20~25 PD. For older patients, reduction in the hyperopic correction may result in accommodative asthenopia, and alternative treatments may be needed.

14.3.3.4 Infantile esotropia and exotropia

Once the diagnosis of infantile esotropia has been confirmed, the clinician should make an effort to determine whether a *superimposed* accommodative component exists, by evaluating the effect of correcting the hyperopic refractive error on the angle of deviation. In most cases, a large esotropia persists, despite corrective lenses, and repeated cycloplegic refractions show little change in the amount of hyperopia. Amblyopia, if present, should be treated. When amblyopia is suspected in preverbal patients who show strong fixation preference, *occlusion therapy* may be used until an alternating fixation pattern is established. The acquisition of alternating fixation implies resolution of amblyopia and should also prevent amblyopia regression. Two hours of daily occlusion of the preferred eye can be prescribed initially. When the esotropia is large and nonaccommodative, surgical ocular alignment should be considered. Most ophthalmic surgeons prefer to intervene before 24 months of age, some as early as 6 months, in the hope of establishing binocular vision. Approximately 40% of treated cases of infantile esotropia achieve some stereopsis. Multiple surgical procedures are frequently needed in such cases.

14.3.3.5 Intermittent exotropia

Individual cases of intermittent exotropia are treated in different ways and often by a combination of treatments. Therapy for intermittent exotropia should include correction of significant refractive error. Usually, the full amount of myopia, anisometropia, and astigmatism should be fully corrected. Hyperopia may be undercorrected for younger patients. Added minus lens power may be used temporarily to help facilitate fusion in children with divergence excess or basic intermittent exotropia. *Compensatory* base-in prisms can be used to facilitate fusion. Numerous vision therapy procedures, including but not limited to expanding fusional vergence amplitudes and vergence facility, diplopia awareness, biofeedback, and increasing accommodation are prescribed for small and moderate size deviations. Surgical intervention should be considered when, after a reasonable time, other treatment modalities have not been successful and the deviation persists or increases.

14.3.3.6 Mechanical esotropia and exotropia

The patient with mechanical esotropia or exotropia may need no specific therapy if there is either minimal or no strabismus in the primary position of gaze and the patient does not experience diplopia. For example, treatment for Duane syndrome, which may have secondary tightness of the medial and/or lateral rectus muscle, is generally restricted to cases in which there is an objectionable compensatory head turn, a large angle strabismus in the primary position, extreme elevation or depression of the eye, or extreme retraction of the globe in adduction. Because head-turning is prevalent, amblyopia is uncommon and high-level stereopsis usually exists. Prisms may be prescribed for slight head turns. For large head turns, surgery may be used, but it does not improve the deficient abduction or adduction.

14.3.3.7 Microtropia

Microtropia is a fully adapted strabismus that rarely gives rise to symptoms unless other conditions become superimposed. Its treatment consists mostly of correcting significant refractive errors and any coexisting amblyopia. The use of vision therapy and prisms to establish bifoveal fusion and high-level stereopsis has been successful in selected cases of microtropia.

14.3.3.8 Sensory esotropia and exotropia

Infants diagnosed at birth with sensory esotropia or exotropia due to unilateral congenital cataracts should be surgically treated within the first 2 months of life. Treatment and management may include cataract surgery, optical correction with contact lens, or *intraocular lens implants*, and occlusion therapy for amblyopia. Neutralizing prisms may be prescribed when fusion exists, and, depending upon the size of the deviation, subsequent strabismus surgery may be performed. The attainment of normal binocular vision is generally not a realistic goal. In older children and adults with acquired sensory exotropia due to dense traumatic unilateral cataracts, fusion may be lost if the cataract remains in situ for more than 2 years, despite subsequent cataract extraction, prisms, vision therapy, and strabismus surgery. Therefore, treatment should not be delayed.

14.3.4 Patient Education

The prognosis, advantages, and disadvantages of the various modes of treatment or management should be discussed with the patient and/or the patient's parents, and a plan based on this dialogue should be developed. Patients who suddenly develop strabismus of undetermined etiology should be informed that such an event may be related to a systemic or neurologic disease that would necessitate referral for consultation with, or treatment or management by, another health care provider. It is important for parents of strabismic children to learn about the condition and the child's risks of developing amblyopia and impaired binocular *depth perception*. Treatment and management plans formulated in consultation with the patient and parents should be responsive to their preferences. The optometrist should elicit the child's and/or the parents' expectations for outcomes, advise the persons involved, relate the findings, prepare treatment and management plans, discuss options, and recommend strategies for successful treatment and management. Parents and children must understand that timely examination and management are critical to reducing the risk for loss of vision and fusion and the development of other symptoms associated with strabismus.

14.4 NYSTAGMUS

14.4.1 Etiology

It occurs due to disturbance of the factors responsible for maintaining normal *ocular posture*. These include disorders of sensory visual pathway, *vestibular apparatus*, *semicircular canals*, mid-brain and *cerebellum*.

14.4.2 Features of Nystagmus

It may be characterized by any of the following features: It may be pendular or jerk nystagmus. In *pendular nystagmus* movements are of equal velocity in each direction. It may be horizontal, vertical or rotatory. In *jerk nystagmus*, the movements have a slow component in one direction and a fast component in the other direction. The direction of jerk nystagmus is defined by direction of the fast component (phase). It may be right, left, up, down or rotatory. Nystagmus movements may be rapid or slow. The movements may be fine or *coarse*. Nystagmus may be latent or manifest.

14.4.3 Types of Nystagmus
14.4.3.1 Physiological nystagmus

1) Optokinetic nystagmus

It is a physiological jerk nystagmus induced by presenting to gaze the objects moving serially in one direction, such as strips of a spinning optokinetic drum. The eyes will follow a fixed strip momentarily and then jerk back to reposition centrally to fix up a new strip.

Similar condition occurs while looking at outside things from a moving train.

2) End-point nystagmus

It is a fine jerk horizontal nystagmus seen in normal persons on extreme right or left gaze.

3) Physiological vestibular nystagmus

It is a jerk nystagmus which can be elicited by stimulating the *tympanic membrane* with hot or cold water. It forms the basis of caloric test. If cold water is poured into right ear the patient develops left jerk nystagmus (rapid phase towards left), while the reverse happens with warm water, i.e., patient develops right jerk nystagmus. It can be remembered by the mnemonic "COWS" (Cold–Opposite, Warm–Same).

14.4.3.2 Sensory deprivation (ocular) nystagmus

1) Congenital pendular (ocular) nystagmus

It is a horizontal slow pendular nystagmus usually associated with sensory deprivation due to reduced central visual acuity. Its common causes are congenital cataract, congenital *toxoplasmosis*, macular *hypoplasia*, aniridia, albinism, optic nerve hypoplasia and *Leber's congenital amaurosis*.

2) Acquired ocular nystagmus

It occurs in monocular adults when they develop decreased visual acuity in the only seeing eye. It is a pendular nystagmus.

3) Miner's nystagmus

It is a rapid rotatory type of nystagmus which occurs in coal mine workers. It probably results from fixation difficulties in the dim illumination.

14.4.3.3 Motor imbalance nystagmus

1) Congenital jerk nystagmus

It is a *hereditary* nystagmus of unknown etiology which persists throughout life. It is *bilateral*, horizontal jerk nystagmus with rapid phase towards the lateral side. It is not present during sleep.

2) Latent nystagmus

It is not present when both eyes are open. It appears when one eye is covered. It is a jerk nystagmus with rapid phase towards the uncovered eye.

3) Spasmus nutans

It is characterised by fine pendular horizontal nystagmus associated with head nodding and abnormal head posture. It appears in infancy and self-resolves by the age of 3 years.

4) Peripheral vestibular nystagmus

It occurs due to diseases of the eighth nerve or vestibular end organ. The nystagmus is jerky, fine, rapid and horizontal-rotatory.

5) Central vestibular nystagmus

It may be of the following types: upbeat nystagmus; down beat nystagmus; periodic alternative nystagmus.

6) Gaze-paretic nystagmus

It is a slow horizontal jerk nystagmus due to upper brain stem dysfunction.

7) Convergence retraction nystagmus

It is a jerk nystagmus with bilateral fast component towards the medial side. It is associated with retraction of the globe in convergence.

8) See-saw nystagmus

In it, one eye rises up and intorts, while the other shifts down and extorts. It is usually associated with upper brain stem *lesions*.

9) Nystagmus blockage syndrome

It is a rare condition in which sudden esotropia develops in infancy to dampen the horizontal nystagmus.

14.4.4 Nystagmus Movements

There are ocular movements which mimic nystagmus. These include:

- *Ocular flutter*, occurs due to interruption of cerebellar connection to brain stem. It is characterized by horizontal oscillation and inability to fixate after change of gaze.
- Opsoclonus, refers to combined horizontal, vertical and/or torsional oscillations associated with *myoclonic* movement of face, arms and legs. It is seen in patients with *encephalitis*.
- Superior oblique *myokymia*, is characterized by monocular, rapid, intermittent, torsional vertical movements (which are best seen on *slit-lamp examination*).
- Ocular bobbing, refers to rapid downward deviation of the eyes with slow up-drift. It occurs due to *pontine* dysfunctions.

14.4.5 Management for Nystagmus

Congenital nystagmus has long been viewed as untreatable, but medications have been discovered in recent years that show promise in some patients. In 1980, researchers discovered that a drug called baclofen could stop periodic alternating nystagmus. Subsequently, gabapentin, an anticonvulsant, led to improvement in about half the patients who took it. Several therapeutic approaches, such as contact lenses, drugs, surgery, and *low vision rehabilitation* have also been proposed. For example, it has been proposed that *mini-telescopic eyeglasses* suppress nystagmus.

Surgical treatment of congenital nystagmus is aimed at improving head posture, simulating *artificial* divergence, or weakening the horizontal recti muscles. Clinical trials of a surgery to treat nystagmus (known as tenotomy) concluded in 2001. Tenotomy is now being performed regularly at numerous centers around the world. The surgery aims to reduce the eye oscillations, which in turn tends to improve visual acuity.

Chapter 15
Low Vision and Vision Rehabilitation

INTRODUCTION
- Visual Impairment Definition and Classification
- Common Causes of Visual Impairment
- Prevalence of Visual Impairment
- Visual Rehabilitation

PATIENT INTERVIEW
- Mental State
- Interview Procedure

REFRACTION AND VISUAL ACUITY MEASUREMENT
- Refraction
- Visual Acuity Measurement

VISUAL FUNCTION ASSESSMENT
- Ocular Health Examination
- Visual Field
- Contrast Sensitivity
- Color Vision

MAGNIFICATION
- Definition of Magnification
- Enlargement Methods
- Low-Vision Aids for Distance
- Low-Vision Aids for Near Vision

NON-OPTICAL AIDS
- Illumination
- Relative Size Enlargement
- Increased Visibility
- Auditory and Tactile Training
- Visual Field Enhancement

15.1 INTRODUCTION

15.1.1 Visual Impairment Definition and Classification

Visual impairment is the loss of *visual acuity* or *visual field*. It encompasses low vision and blindness and can be defined as vision that is not adequate for the patient's needs.

Blindness standards are different in different countries. In China, we define visual acuity equal to or worse than 0.05 (*decimal* visual acuity) in the better-seeing eye or a visual field equal to or less than 10 degrees in the widest meridian of the better-seeing eye as being legally blind. In the United States and the United Kingdom, the visual field is limited to $\leqq 20$ degrees, and the visual acuity of the better-seeing eye is $\leqq 6/60$ in the United States and $\leqq 6/120$ in the United Kingdom. The World Health Organization defines visual acuity as a visual acuity $\leqq 6/120$ in the better-seeing eye and a visual field less than 10 degrees in the widest meridian of the better-seeing eye.

In 2003, the World Health Organization proposed that visual impairment can be divided into mild, moderate and severe. Visual acuity between 6/12 and 6/18 indicates mild visual impairment, between 6/18 and 6/60 indicates moderate visual impairment, and between 6/60 and 3/60 indicates severe visual impairment. In 2018, the international classification of diseases classified visual impairment into two groups: distance and near. For near visual impairment, the definition is near visual acuity worse than N6 at 40 cm, which equals 0.3 around decimal visual acuity.

15.1.2 Common Causes of Visual Impairment

Many diseases can cause visual impairment, such as uncorrected refractive error, cataracts, *age-related macular degeneration*, glaucoma, *diabetic retinopathy*, corneal opacity, *trachomo*, albinism, *retinitis pigmentosa*, aniridia, rod *monochromatism*, Stargardt's maculopathy, Lebers congenital amaurosis, cone-rod dystrophies, retinal *coloboma*, microphthalmos, optic atrophy, optic nerve hypoplasia, congenital nystagmus, *retinopathy of prematurity* and some syndromes.

Among them, uncorrected refractive error and untreated cataract are the two most common causes of visual impairment in middle- and low-income countries, whereas age-related macular degeneration and glaucoma are the two most common causes of visual impairment in developed countries. In children, the most common causes are *hereditary disorders*. Different diseases typically differ in terms of occurrence and development, which will affect the development of appropriate treatment strategies.

15.1.3 Prevalence of Visual Impairment

There are at least 2.2 billion people who have visual impairment worldwide, and at least half of these cases could have been prevented or have yet to be addressed. Most people with vision impairment are over 50 years old. There are an estimated 6.7 million people with blindness in China, and the prevalence of blindness is approximately 0.6%. The regional blindness burden is the percentage of the world's blind population living within a region of interest, and it is approximately 0.82. There are 0.45 million people newly diagnosed with blindness and 1.35 million people newly diagnosed with low vision every year in China. Additionally, there will be 3 patients newly diagnosed with low vision and 1 patient newly diagnosed with blindness every minute. The developed industrialized nations have approximately 2.4 million blind people, and the regional prevalence of blindness is approximately 0.3%.

15.1.4 Visual Rehabilitation

When assessing a visually impaired patient, we need to assess their visual rehabilitation needs, ocular health and visual functions, which include visual acuity, refraction, *contrast sensitivity*, visual field, glare evaluation, color vision test and dark/light adaptation. The impact on development or day-to-day life is *enormous*.

The overall goal of vision rehabilitation is to recapture, strengthen and maintain self-confidence for safe, dependency functions, maximize the use of any *residual vision*, and enhance an individual's functional ability independence in daily living. *Rehabilitation training*, such as *orientation* and *mobility* rehabilitation, is just as vital as choosing low-vision devices. Orientation refers to awareness of the environment or surroundings. This type of rehabilitation can help patients learn training techniques, search patterns, and sighted guide techniques and can aid with independent travel in a variety of environments. White *cane* is the most widely used technique; a person *wielding* a white cane indicates that they are visually impaired. In addition to low-vision optometrists, there are many other blind or low-vision professions, such as vision rehabilitation therapists, teachers of visually impaired individuals, low-vision rehabilitation therapists and orientation and mobility specialists. They all collaborate to aid in the rehabilitation of visually impaired patients.

15.2 PATIENT INTERVIEW

15.2.1 Mental State

Patients with low vision are usually accompanied by a period of abnormal *mental* state because of their visual impairment. According to previous studies, there are five stages of the emotional response to loss: denial, anger, bargaining, depression and acceptance (coexistence). The duration of each stage is affected by the *severity* and onset age of visual impairment, acute or *chronic* visual loss, understanding of the diagnosis, prognosis expectations, and personality. Furthermore, patients at various stages can have vastly varied reactions to clinicians. We must pay close attention to patients' mental states and have suitable communication methods in the clinic. If there are problems with an abnormal mental state, a *psychologist* should be consulted without delay.

15.2.2 Interview Procedure

The low-vision clinic actually begins before we greet the patients. Based on the different stages in which we communicate with patients with low vision, we divide the interview procedure into 3 steps: before the clinic, greeting and observing, and case history.

15.2.2.1 Before the clinic

After patients with low vision or their families make appointments, social workers initiate contact with all new patients by phone, as we need to know the basic information before the clinic appointment starts. Social workers usually collect information about the names of the eye conditions and past and present eye care, which includes the treatment accepted, the low-vision *aids* used, the current functional use of vision and goals for clinical evaluation. The patients need to bring all their glasses, even if they are not helping, as well as all low-vision devices they have ever used and any previous eye reports. All these steps can provide information on a patient's eye health and previous therapy, such as low-vision aids or low-vision rehabilitation.

Moreover, we need to know about patients' general health conditions and the medications they take. Many patients and their families may not have a very *comprehensive* understanding of their general health; therefore, we usually advise them to prepare a list of medications.

The clinic appointment will be guided by knowing what patients expect from this clinic visit. Patients may have different goals, and some of them have several goals. We can ask them to write down and list their goals. They can also bring specialized goal-related materials, such as schoolwork, textbooks, newspapers, crafts and work materials.

15.2.2.2 Greeting and observing

Unlike the ordinary clinic, we like to go out to the waiting area to greet the patients. By greeting patients in the waiting room, we can decrease patients' *apprehension* and observe their behavior at the same time. Because of their low visual acuity, it is often better to greet the patients by shaking their hands and performing self-introduction to let the patients feel us in case they cannot see our faces clearly. Finally, please do not forget to ask "Do you need assistance to go to the clinic room?" We are reminded to constantly consider the patient's low visual acuity.

When we see patients in the waiting room, we should observe each patient's interactions with others, interactions with the environment, appearance abnormalities, and postural abnormalities, along with other behaviors. According to these abnormalities, we can obtain *clues* about their visual conditions and psychological conditions. After some visual problems persist for a period of time, patients can regain their compensatory position to achieve better visual acuity or a better visual field. If we can find these abnormal postures, we can obtain some disease clues. For example, if a patient has left-sided *hemianopsia*, they usually form a right-sided head turn *involuntarily*. If the patient shows a head *tilt*, the cause can be *photophobia* or severe glare bother.

15.2.2.3 Case history

A comprehensive case history collection is critical because it allows clinicians to compile a list of reference information and quickly locate what is most significant. The following is an example of a typical case history:

- General data: Patient name, sex, age, nationality, and source of history.
- *Chief complaint* (cc): A short sentence reflecting the main problem. For example, I cannot read newspapers now.
- *History of present illness* (HPI): A paragraph explaining the chief complaint in detail should usually be recorded following the timeline.
- *Past medical history* (PMH): The important medical condition of the whole body, including prevention, diagnosis and treatment, in the past.
- *Medications* and *allergies*: Any type of medication the patient is taking now and any types of allergies known, including food, medications, and the environment.
- Family history: Any family member who has general problems or eye problems, such as cancer, *hypertension*, diabetes, blindness, glaucoma, and age-related macular degeneration.
- Systemic review: A systemic review of what we talked about before and a supplement to the missing items.

For patients with low vision, we need to pay more attention to their eye condition and daily life situation, including the following:

- Ocular symptoms: Are there any *fluctuations*, glare, or dark or light adaptation issues?
- Vocation history: Current status, type of work, and functional aspects of joy.
- Educational history: Current educational status, highest grade completed, issues in school, services received in school, favorite subject, and least favorite subject.
- Visual concern: Any problems or concerns about reading, mobility, activities of daily living, education issues, or vocational issues.

In addition to comprehensive case history collection, goal orientation is also very important. Each patient has individual goals, and patients' goals guide our low-vision evaluation. Good goals should be *concrete*, *realistic*, and positive, and when utilizing techniques and devices, success should be demonstrated. Moreover, good goal setting can help motivate patients toward success.

15.3 REFRACTION AND VISUAL ACUITY MEASUREMENT

Providing patients with appropriate refraction and correction can improve patients' visual acuity, and the target visual acuity magnification could decrease. A lower magnification needs to equal a larger valid visual field, which is a lighter and more convenient low-vision aid.

15.3.1 Refraction

Low-vision refraction is usually more complex. The patients could have scars on their cornea or retina, they could have *eccentric* viewing, the *refracting media* could be opaque, and the patients might not respond well. When refraction is performed on patients with low vision, we can use an automatic refractor or retinoscopy to obtain an initial refractive error.

15.3.1.1 Objective refraction

In low-vision refraction, we usually do not use phoropters because the use of a phoropter blocks our view to observe patients' ocular movement, viewing, and distance between their eyes and the phoropter. Additionally, some patients with low vision have compensatory eye positions, so the use of phoropters limits their head or eye movements. In that way, low-vision refraction is best performed "the old-fashioned way" with a *trial frame* and loose lenses. Using a trail frame can help us maintain a more consistent distance between our lenses and eyes. Moreover, changing refractive lens power always requires a larger range in patients with low vision. Using a trail frame allows clinicians to incorporate other lenses to demonstrate to patients.

15.3.1.2 Subjective refraction

After the initial refraction diopter is obtained, we need to perform subjective refraction, which requires the patient's response. Most patients with low vision are unable to notice small power changes. Therefore, how can a proper power change be chosen to allow comparisons of subjective refraction? Researchers have reported that using the "just noticeable difference" (JND) diopter can achieve the best effect; it is the smallest increment in the change in lens power that can just be noticed by the patient. The "just noticeable difference" can be obtained by *calculating* the best corrected visual acuity at present and converting it to a 10-foot test distance. The *denominator divided by* 100 is the JND power. Specifically, if the patient's corrected visual acuity is 20/400 on the ETDRS (The early treatment diabetic retinopathy study) visual acuity chart at present, we convert it to a 10-foot test distance, which should be 10/200 visual acuity. Therefore, we should take 2.00 D as the JND lens and show the patient +2.00 D and −2.00 D lenses. If the patient was +2.00 D, we place the +2.00 D in the frame and check the visual acuity again. We should pay attention to modifying JND power along with visual acuity changes.

15.3.2 Visual Acuity Measurement

15.3.2.1 Visual acuity chart

When testing distance/near visual acuity in patients with low vision, there are some typical specificities that we need to know. First, not every patient can read the visual acuity chart. For infants, toddlers, and those who cannot cooperate, other exam methods are needed.

Visual acuity is a *dynamic* functional indicator that is affected by the test environment, illumination, optotype contrast, and patients' attention and communication. Considering vision loss, we usually use a moveable visual acuity chart. If patients cannot see the first row at the normal test distance, we can move the visual acuity chart closer.

There are several types of distance visual acuity charts, such as the Bailey-Lovie Chart, the ETDRS Chart (Early Treatment of Diabetic Retinopathy), and the Lea Chart. A good visual acuity chart should have the same task at each level, which means that the letter size should be the only significant variable from one level to the next. This requires that there should be the same number of letters at each size level, that the spacing between letters and between rows should be proportional to the letter size, and that the letters should be balanced for *legibility* and *logarithmic* size progression (constant ratio). For distance visual acuity measurements, we recommend the use of the ETDRS Chart.

For near visual acuity testing, there are several charts, such as the Bailey-Lovie word reading chart, the MN read chart, the Sloan M chart, and the Jaeger Notation. Above all, the near visual acuity charts can be roughly divided into continuous texts and single-letter charts. In fact, reading words or text is a more complex task than reading spaced letters in patients with low vision. Even if patients do not need to see every letter clearly, reading words or text is a more realistic way to test them, as it is closer to patients' daily lives.

15.3.2.2 Illumination

The illumination should be adjustable because some diseases affect light visual acuity more, whereas other diseases may affect dim visual acuity more. Moreover, even at different ambient illumination levels, we need a high-contrast visual acuity chart. Patients with low vision have decreased contrast sensitivity.

15.3.2.3 Procedure

Importantly, we need to begin testing visual acuity with an "easy" condition. Performance is usually evaluated at thresholds and suprathreshold. In that way, patients can achieve success and gain confidence. They will be more motivated to participate in the test and more motivated to respond. If the chart is initially held close, expecting poor acuity performance, and if the patient does much better than expected, it will be easy to then move the chart to a farther distance. When testing and recording visual acuity, we do not recommend using "hand move" or "count fingers" assessments. One reason is that if patients see an actual letter, they will feel much more confident than if they just see fingers or hands, even at extremely close distances. Moreover, obtaining a specific number will help us calculate the following magnification and choose low-vision aids.

When testing a patient's distance visual acuity, we need to test both monocular and binocular acuity and usually start with easy tasks. If the patient has a compensatory eye or head position, we can let him or her use the best way to perform the test and record it. The most commonly used distance visual acuity recording is Snellen. The numerator in the Snellen visual acuity recording is the testing distance, and the denominator is the letter size that you can see.

For near visual acuity, we always ask patients to hold the chart wherever they want. Because patients with low vision usually do not have sufficient accommodation, we should add additional power when testing near visual acuity. Typically, the test chart has a normal and a reversed model, which has a black background with white words. We can let the patient choose which one is better and then use that one to test. To record near visual acuity, we always use the M system, where 1 M equals 12 font size letters. Similarly, if the patient can read 1 M size letter at approximately 0.5 m, we record the visual acuity as 0.5/1 M, which is approximately equivalent to 20/50 at 0.5 m. Notably, the endpoint is important. It is not the words or texts patients cannot read at all. The endpoint should be the words or texts patients read markedly more slowly than before. However, tasks are more standardized and the difficulties are more uniform with the word reading chart.

15.4 VISUAL FUNCTION ASSESSMENT

15.4.1 Ocular Health Examination

Although patients with low vision have always had comprehensive clinic experiences previously, an ocular health exam remains a top priority. We still utilize a slit lamp to examine the patient's eye lids, lashes, conjunctiva, cornea, anterior chamber, anterior chamber angle, iris, lens, and intraocular pressure at the beginning of the low-vision clinic. We then use a digital wide-field lens or ophthalmoscopy to examine the vitreous and retina. Additionally, we need to perform a light test on the pupils, observe the pupils' size and shape, compare the two pupils, and observe whether the light reflex is normal. After that, we need to perform Hirschberg and cover tests to examine the patient's eye alignment. Following the eye movement test, we need to examine whether the eye movements are smooth and sufficient.

15.4.2 Visual Field

There are two types of visual field examinations: *static* visual field examination and dynamic visual field examination. Common visual field examination methods include the Amsler Grid, *confrontation visual field,* automated static threshold *perimetry,* manual kinetic perimetry, and functional visual field methods. We need to judge the proper method to test each patient's visual field. When we want to assess the patient's condition with the most accuracy and they can cooperate, automated static threshold perimetry, such as Humphrey or Octopus, can be used. Machines can provide a more precise result, but they require better cooperation and visual acuity.

Mostly, when we need a rough approximation of the patient's visual field just in the clinic, we often use the Amsler Grid or a confrontation visual field. The Amsler grid is a quick way to test where there is any kind of missing data or distortion in the central 10-degree visual field. The confrontation visual field test is also widely used in the clinic, especially for those who cannot respond well to machines. As when performing visual field confrontation, we compare a patient's visual field edges with our own, it can be easily determined whether general defects are present.

15.4.3 Contrast Sensitivity

Contrast sensitivity measures a patient's ability to detect *subtle* differences between light and dark objects at a given distance. Patients with low vision usually also have decreased contrast sensitivity. There are many low-contrast visual tasks in daily life, such as curbs, stairs, and faces.

Reduced contrast sensitivity is easier to measure than treated contrast sensitivity. In the clinic, we can use the Vector vision contrast sensitivity chart, the Pelli-Robson chart, the CamBlobs, and the Mars numeral contrast sensitivity test.

15.4.3.1 Mars numeral contrast sensitivity

Among them, the Mars numeral contrast sensitivity test is most widely used. It is a set of charts for testing the threshold contrast sensitivity that patients can detect. When we use the Mars numeral contrast sensitivity test, we should test with the light on, and the *optimal luminance* should be 85 cd/m^2. Additionally, unlike visual acuity tests, contrast sensitivity tests require a certain range of testing distances, usually between 30 cm and 50 cm. Because this test is an assessment of near visual acuity, we need to provide a somewhat positive addition to ensure that there is enough accommodation. If patients hold the chart too closely, the results will be overestimated. There are three charts in the Mars numeral contrast sensitivity test: one for the right eye, one for the left eye, and the other for binocular testing. When the test begins, the patient is requested to read the letters in order. We need to record the number of errors. Two kinds of endpoints are admitted: one is that the patient reads two continuous letters incorrectly. The other is that even if we encourage the patient, he still fails to read the following letters.

The calculation is the final log contrast sensitivity = log contrast sensitivity value at the final correct letter − number of errors prior to the final correct letter × 0.04. The grading is profound (<0.48), severe (0.52~1.00), moderate (1.04~1.48) or normal.

15.4.3.2 Contrast sensitivity measurement for young children

For those who cannot read the Mars numeral contrast sensitivity test, such as young children or infants, there are specially designed contrast sensitivity tests: the Hiding Heidi low contrast face test, the Berkeley disc test, the Mr. Happy contrast test, and the Lighthouse contrast sensitivity chart. All of them use shapes, leaf symbols or faces to simplify patients' responses. The Hiding Heidi and Mr. Happy tests use the force choice method. We just need to judge the patient's preferential looking side. The Lighthouse chart requests that patients identify or match symbols at each contrast level.

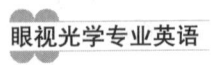

15.4.4 Color Vision

Color vision defects can be classified as acquired or hereditary color vision loss. Hereditary color vision defects are usually binocular and static, and patients always have normal visual acuity, contrast sensitivity and visual fields. Conversely, acquired color vision defects are usually monocular and asymmetric, often progressive and have abnormal visual acuity, contrast sensitivity or visual field. Any defect affecting the optic nerve or cones can cause acquired color vision defects, such as optic nerve atrophy, macular damage, cone dystrophy, and the late stage of *retinitis pigmentosa*.

15.4.4.1 Red comparison

Among these conditions, patients with optic nerve diseases are always sensitive to red color. The perception of red will fade away in the damaged eye. Therefore, a quick test is needed to determine whether there is an optic nerve problem by asking patients to compare a red eye drop cap.

15.4.4.2 D-15 test

Because of visual acuity requests, patients with low vision cannot use the same test books as normal patients can. At least 20/200 visual acuity is required for the Ishihara test book. Even patients with visual acuity better than 20/200 are not recommended because the visual task is too *crowded* to recognize for patients with low vision.

An enlarged version of the D-15 test is the best method for testing elderly children and adults. The D-15 test has relatively high contrast sensitivity, a lower requirement of visual acuity and an easy visual processing procedure.

15.4.4.3 Color vision measurement for young children

For young children who cannot handle the D-15 test, there are still forced-choice preferential-looking tests, such as the Color naming test, Color matching test and PACT plates test. Finally, every type of test should be tested with normal illumination.

15.5 MAGNIFICATION

Magnification is the ratio of retinal image heights with and without magnification. The *calculation formula* is that magnification equals the angular height of an object viewed through a magnifier divided by the angular height of the object measured at the eye. Typically, four types of magnification are used:
- Apparent magnification;
- Relative magnification;
- Iso-accommodative magnification;
- Trade magnification.

15.5.1 Definition of Magnification

Apparent magnification, also called perceived magnification or angular magnification, is the ratio of the angle that the image subtends the pupil to the angle that the object subtends the pupil. It is compared with and without a *magnifier*.

Relative magnification compares the viewing with a magnifier to a standard viewing situation, which is usually at 25 cm. It is the ratio of the angle that the image subtends at the pupil to the angle that the object subtends at a distance of 25 cm.

Iso-accommodative magnification is the ratio of the angle that the image subtends at a specified distance from the pupil to the angle that the object subtends at the same distance.

Trade magnification is a special case of iso-accommodative magnification. It is the ratio of the angle that the image subtends at 25 cm from the pupil to the angle that the object subtends at 25 cm. Different types of magnification are always used for different habits and needs.

15.5.2 Enlargement Methods

To achieve magnification, there are four commonly used enlargement methods in patients with low vision:
- Relative distance enlargement;
- Relative size enlargement;
- Electronic enlargement;
- Angular enlargement.

Relative distance enlargement results from a reduction in the object viewing distance. In that way, we can increase the angular subtense of the object when it is viewed at a new working distance. This approach is the easiest way to achieve enlargement, and many patients can use relative distance enlargement by themselves involuntarily. Moreover, many visually impaired patients do not have sufficient accommodation. Therefore, when the relative distance is increased, the patient should be given corresponding accommodations to ensure successful and prolonged use. When patients hold their materials closer, their efficient visual field decreases.

Relative size enlargement increases the size of the object while the working distance remains the same. It is provided by nonoptic aids, such as large print books.

Project enlargement involves projecting or electronically changing the image form to obtain an increased angular subtend of a new image. The most commonly used system is the electronic vision enhancement system (EVES). When an EVES is used, patients can obtain not only magnification but also better contrast sensitivity.

Angular enlargement is the ratio of the angle subtended by the image through the optical system to the angle subtended by the object when viewed directly. The vergence of light passing through the optic system may be unchanged. The most representative low-vision aids with angular enlargement are *telescopic* aids. If the patient is given more than one enlargement, the total magnification should be combined.

15.5.3 Low-Vision Aids for Distance

In the low-vision clinic, we should consider providing distance magnification for a patient with goals such as seeing road signs or watching TV. When trying to achieve a patient's distance visual tasks, what we must have is the patient's best corrected visual acuity and target visual acuity (which comes from the patient's goals). In addition, the functional visual field, contrast sensitivity, illumination, and the patient's skills and coordination should also be considered.

The magnification we need to use is the ratio of the patient's best corrected visual acuity (the better-seeing eye) to the target visual acuity. If the patient's best corrected visual acuity is 20/200 and the target acuity is 20/40, then we need to ideally use 5x magnification. To achieve magnification to achieve distance target visual acuity, there are *telescopes* (hand-held telescopes, clip-on telescopes, spectacle telescopes, full diameter telescopes, bioptic telescopes, surgical telescopes), CCTVs and cutting-edge electronic low-vision aids from which to choose.

Telescopes are lens systems that improve the resolution of distance objects through enlargement of the retinal image and can be divided into Galilean and Keplerian telescopes. In a *Keplerian telescope*, the objective and ocular lenses are both convex lenses, whereas in a *Galilean telescope*, the objective lens is a convex lens and the eyepiece is a concave lens. A Keplerian telescope usually has an *inverted image* and is longer, heavier, and has higher magnification. Conversely, the Galileo telescope is a shorter, lighter, lower-magnification telescope that produces an *erect image*.

15.5.4 Low-Vision Aids for Near Vision

When talking about near vision magnifiers, the first thing we should keep in mind is that testing distance is the most important consideration in the whole procedure. The M system is the most commonly used visual acuity system in near vision magnifiers. In the M system, when the patient holds a visual chart 0.5 m away from his or her eyes and can read a 2 M size letter, we record his or her visual acuity as 0.5/2 M.

15.5.4.1 Equivalent viewing distance and equivalent viewing power

When calculating the near magnification, we use two concepts: the equivalent viewing distance (EVD) and the equivalent viewing power (EVP). The equivalent viewing distance is the distance at which the object subtends an angle that is equal to the angle the image subtends at the eye. The EVD is equal to the eye-to-image distance divided by the enlargement ratio. The equivalent viewing power is the *reciprocal* of EVD.

15.5.4.2 Calculation of the magnification

Equivalent viewing power is most commonly used when a near visual magnifier is used. The best corrected near visual acuity and target acuity are still two items we must know when performing the near visual magnification calculation. Another factor of the same importance is the working distance. We can use the same method as distance to calculate the enlargement ratio, which should be the target visual acuity divided by the best corrected visual acuity. Then, the testing distance is divided by the enlargement ratio to obtain the equivalent viewing distance. The reciprocal is used to obtain the equivalent viewing power. For example, if the patient's best corrected near visual acuity is 0.4/4 M, the target is to see the 1 M letter size book. We obtained an enlargement ratio of 4 M/1 M, which was equal to 4. Because the near visual acuity testing distance is 0.5 m, the EVD should be 0.4 m/4, which equals 0.1 m. The EVP should be 1/0.1 m, which equals +10 D. Therefore, to achieve the target, we need to give the near magnifiers approximately +10 D.

15.5.4.3 Low vision aids for near magnification

For near magnification devices, *microscopes*, hand-held magnifiers, stand magnifiers, telemicroscopes, and electronic magnification systems can also be used. Among them, microscopes utilize the principle of relative distance enlargement, which is the most familiar method for patients and produces the largest field of view. A telemicroscope is a combination of a telescope and a microscope. It uses a plus lens placed over the objective lens of the telescope. The equivalent viewing power of the telemicroscope is the telescope magnification times the dioptric power of the reading cap. Importantly, the recommended reading distance should be the reciprocal of the reading cap diopter. For example, a 20 D telemicroscope can be a 5x telescope with a +4 D reading cap that reads 25 cm away. It can also be a 10x telescope with a +2 D reading cap, reading 50 cm away. A telemicroscope can provide magnification over a wide range and has a wide variety of available equivalent powers.

15.6 NON-OPTICAL AIDS

Non-optical aids are methods that we use to maximize residual visual potential without the use of optical devices; they are typically classified in terms of illumination and contrast sensitivity, glare, relative size magnification, *auditory*, and *tactus*.

15.6.1 Illumination

Lighting has been shown to have significant effects on both mobility and reading. Illumination is defined as the amount of light falling on an object or surface. Increased aging requires increased illumination due to the loss of light *transmittance* and light *scatter* of short wavelengths. Lighting can have the greatest impact on cataracts and macular changes. An older person needs approximately 3~4 times as much light as a young person needs for the lighting to be sufficient.

The intensity of light falling on an object is proportional to the intensity of the source and the reciprocal of the distance squared. Therefore, when the light distance is closer to the object surface, there will be more illumination. Owing to the cosine law of the light intensity formula, we obtain the strongest light intensity when the light is perpendicular.

Patients with low vision have different pathologies and different goals; therefore, it is important to perform lighting evaluations. We can focus on those goals and their own environments. A home environment lighting assessment is a questionnaire that can capture detailed light situations and the patient's needs. A higher light intensity can always provide patients with better contrast sensitivity. Most visually impaired patients are affected by a decrease in contrast sensitivity. Enhancing lighting is the easiest way to improve contrast sensitivity. Moreover, contrast sensitivity can be *optimized* by using plain backgrounds with a contrasting foreground, such as black writing on a white page. We can use different color combinations to ask patients to compare and choose the most comfortable reading one to provide.

There are difficulties in how to balance the amount of compensated light to help enhance contrast sensitivity without exacerbating glare. Every eye disease can cause glare issues, such as maculopathies, optic neuropathies, retinal dystrophies, cataracts, corneal opacities, and traumatic brain injuries. Glare control is important to minimize glare discomfort or disability by controlling the amount of light entering the eyes. We can provide antiglare tinted lenses or filters to control glare. There are many kinds of tinted colors, and multiple tints always need to be evaluated under conditions where the patient is experiencing light sensitivity. *Additionally, antireflective coatings* on glasses can eliminate reflections of light from the front and back surfaces of the lenses, which can improve not only the impact of light but also the appearance of the patient's glasses. Because most of the glare is from horizontal surfaces, *polarizers* can also be oriented to block that radiation. Notably, reversing polarity is a useful way to control glare and enhance contrast sensitivity in some patients. When reversing the polarity, which means that we use a black background and white words, it can help to remove the glare of the white background.

15.6.2 Relative Size Enlargement

Another commonly used non-optical strategy is relative size enlargement method, which included large print books, bold and raised line papers, bold markers, and writing guides. If the patient's magnification needs are not high, relative size enlargement can be achieved. If the relative size enlargement is not enough, it can also result in less magnification needed, which means a greater field of view.

15.6.3 Increased Visibility

In addition to relative size enlargement, there are many other methods, such as increased visibility, supplementary lighting or additional contrasts, alternative outputs that stimulate the nonvisual senses, safety modifications to avoid nonsafe tasks, and appliances with modifications designed to assist anyone with physical infirmity.

In daily life, many situations in which a non-optical strategy can be used exist. In the kitchen, increasing safety is a key issue because everyday living requires the use of knives, matches, cookers and hot food or liquids. We can use liquid level indicators, easy-to-see timers, food slicers, chopping boards and knives, plate surrounds, and talking microwaves and scales. When writing, the use of non-optical aids can assist in keeping the writing straight and increasing the visibility of the print by enhancing the contrast using writing frames, thick or raised lined paper, or a black pen on white paper. *Typoscopes*, which are usually black cards or plastic sheets with a section removed, can be placed as an overlay and thus reduce the glare from the page and assist with the task of keeping to a straight line or finding the appropriate section on a piece of paper. For travel and mobility, we provide canes to help patients.

15.6.4 Auditory and Tactile Training

For those who are severely visually impaired, vision is not the most functional way of performing tasks. Additionally, in some processing diseases, visual acuity during the final stage is severely impaired. Under these two conditions, we can provide auditory or *tactile* training and help. Text-to-speech devices and audiobooks are available for such patients. Moreover, we can teach them *braille*.

15.6.5 Visual Field Enhancement

One more aspect we want to mention is visual field enhancement. We can divide the types of visual field defects into concentric visual field loss, central vision defects, and hemianopia. These defects can alter a patient's behavior as their reading ability deteriorates; in addition, their mobility can become restricted.

15.6.5.1 Concentric visual field loss

For those with concentric visual field loss, the principle is to move the items in the defect area to the normal area. Then, we can obtain reverse telescopes, *minifiers*, and amorphic lenses. When a person looks through a telescope in the reverse direction, there is an apparent increase in the field of view approximately equal to the power of the telescope. The advantages of reverse telescopes are as follows:
- Provide a significant increase in the visual area seen in the residual field;
- May be used hand-held or spectacle-mounted;
- The image is relatively clear.

There are still several disadvantages:
- Reduces visual acuity by a factor of *minification;*
- Objects appear farther away;
- Can only be used as a spotting device while traveling;
- The field of the telescope limits the area of expansion.

Amorphic lenses are similar to reverse telescopes. The difference is that an amorphic lens just minifies in the horizontal or vertical meridian. In that way, the patient's depth perception and the speed of image movement do not change. The objects will be amorphic in one direction; thus, these lenses can only be used in spot viewing.

15.6.5.2 Hemianopic visual field loss

We usually provide prisms to hemianopic patients to assist them. The basic principle is to use a prism to move the image such that patients can see it to enlarge the residual visual field. Patients can use a prism to spot view as well as to aid with mobility after training. Importantly, the base of the prism should face the visual field direction.

Types of prisms include the Fresnel prism, the Elipeli prism, the Gottlieb prism and the Yorked prism. A Fresnel prism is a 1 mm thick plastic material. It is typically prescribed at 30~40 prism diopters and is applied on the back surface of spectacle lenses. Through a Fresnel prism, image displacement in degrees is equal to approximately half of the dioptric power of the prism. Additionally, the use of a Fresnel prism can decrease image clarity and contrast sensitivity.

A Yorked prism is often used in reading; it starts with a 5 prism diopter for each eye. Additionally, the base of the prism should be toward the field defect and should be oriented in the same direction in both eyes. For example, we provide a base-out prism for the left eye and a base-in prism for the right eye in left hemianopsia patients. Yorked prisms cannot be used to assist with mobility.

15.6.5.3 Central visual field defects

Those with central visual field defects are usually subjected to a combination of magnification and eccentric viewing. An eccentric viewing point must be identified, and then that area should be magnified. Additionally, when any area outside the fovea is used, the contrast must be increased. A facial field or clock face can then be used to train patients in eccentric viewing.

Chapter 16
Binocular Vision

EXTRAOCULAR MUSCLES AND OCULAR MOVEMENT
PHYSIOLOGY OF NORMAL BINOCULAR VISION
- ▶ Retinal Correspondence
- ▶ Fusion
- ▶ Stereopsis

ABNORMALITIES OF BINOCULAR VISION
- ▶ Suppression
- ▶ Amblyopia
- ▶ Confusion
- ▶ Diplopia

16.1 EXTRAOCULAR MUSCLES AND OCULAR MOVEMENT

Six extraocular muscles control the movements of each eye. Rectus muscles are superior rectus (SR), inferior rectus (IR), medial rectus (MR) and lateral rectus (LR). The oblique muscles are superior oblique (SO) and inferior oblique (IO). Primary and secondary actions of each muscle are shown in *Table 16-1*.

Table 16-1 Actions of extraocular muscles

Muscle	Primary	Secondary
MR	Adduction	-
LR	Abduction	-
SR	Elevation	Intorsion and adduction
IR	Depression	Extorsion and adduction
SO	Intorsion	Depression and abduction
IO	Extorsion	Elevation and abduction

There are six types of ocular movements:
- Adduction: Move eyes inward along with the vertical axis.
- Abduction: Move eyes outward along with the vertical axis.
- Elevation: Move eyes upward along with the horizontal axis.
- Depression: Move eyes downward along with the horizontal axis.
- *Intorsion*: Move eyes rotatory medially along the anteroposterior axis.
- Extorsion: Move eyes rotatory laterally along the anteroposterior axis.

For both eyes, there are two types of binocular movement: coordination and vergence. Coordinations are both eyes' movements in the same direction, which are synchronous symmetric movements. In contrast, vergences are synchronous and symmetric movements of both eyes in opposite directions.

16.2 PHYSIOLOGY OF NORMAL BINOCULAR VISION

Without an understanding of the physiology of binocular vision it becomes difficult, not impossible, to appreciate its anomalies. The basic laws of binocular vision and *spatial localization* that were laid down by these giants of the past form the very foundation on which our current understanding of strabismus and its symptoms and sensory consequences is based.

The current tendency is to overemphasize *stereopsis* as the only important reason for having a binocular vision. For instance, except for stereopsis, seeing with both eyes is marginal, if any, better than seeing with one—absolute threshold, differential threshold, and visual acuity being about the same. Binocular *concordant* information provides better exteroception of form and color and better appreciation of the day dynamic relationship of the body to the environment, thereby facilitating control of manipulation, reaching, and balance. Also, the advantages of an intact binocular field of vision, which is larger than a monocular field, and central visual field overlap become obvious as soon as the function of one eye becomes impaired by a disease process. There are three grades of binocular single vision, which are *Grade I — Simultaneous perception, Grade II — Fusion, Grade III — Stereopsis*.

16.2.1 Retinal Correspondence
16.2.1.1 Law of retinal correspondence

Retinal elements of the two eyes that share a common subjective visual direction are called corresponding retinal points. All other retinal elements are non-corresponding or disparate with respect to a given retinal element in the fellow eye. This definition also may be stated in the following way: corresponding retinal elements are those elements of the two retinas that give rise in binocular vision to the localization of sensations in one and the same subjective visual direction. It does not matter whether a stimulus reaches the retinal element in one eye alone or its corresponding partner in the other eye alone or whether it reaches both simultaneously the common visual direction of the fovea is again of special importance. All visual directions, as have been seen, have a relative value in subjective space. The common subjective visual directions, have a fixed position relative only to the principal common visual direction. They determine the orientation of visual objects relative to each other with the principal visual direction as the direction of reference.

Corresponding retinal elements arranged in horizontal and vertical rows provide the subjective vertical and horizontal meridians. Meridians that include the visual direction of the fovea are the principal corresponding horizontal and vertical meridians.

The existence of corresponding retinal elements with their common relative subjective visual directions is the essence of binocular vision. It may be called the law of sensory correspondence in analogy with the law of motor correspondence.

16.2.1.2 Law of sensory correspondence

When we place an object at a distance in front of an observer at eye level and in the midplane of the head, if the eyes are properly aligned and the object is fixated binocularly, an image will be received on matching areas of the two retinas; if the eyes are functioning normally and equally, the two images will be the same in size, illuminance, and color. In spite of the presence of the two separate physical (retinal) images, only one visual object is perceived by the observer. This phenomenon is so natural to us that the naive observer is not surprised by it; he is surprised only if he sees double. Yet the opposite—single binocular vision from two distinct retinal images—is the truly remarkable phenomenon that requires an explanation.

16.2.2 Fusion
16.2.2.1 Sensory fusion

Sensory correspondence explains binocular single vision or sensory fusion. The term is defined as the *unification* of visual excitations from corresponding retinal images into a single visual percept, a single visual image. An object localized in one and the same visual direction by stimulation of the two retinas can only appear as one. An individual cannot see double with corresponding retinal elements. Single vision is the *hallmark* of retinal correspondence. Put otherwise, the stimulus to sensory fusion is the excitation of corresponding retinal elements.

Since both the central and peripheral parts of the retina contribute fusible material, it is misleading to equate sensory fusion with "central" fusion (as opposed to "peripheral" or motor fusion). Fusion, whether sensory or motor, is always a central process (i.e., it takes place in the visual centers of the brain).

For sensory fusion to occur, the images not only must be located on corresponding retinal areas but also must be sufficiently similar in size, brightness, and sharpness. Unequal images are a severe sensory obstacle to fusion. Obstacles to fusion may become important factors in the etiology of strabismus. Differences in color and *contours* may lead to retinal *rivalry.*

The simultaneous stimulation of noncorresponding or disparate retinal elements by an object point causes this point to be localized in two different subjective visual directions. An object point seen simultaneously in two directions appears double or in diplopia. Double vision is the hallmark of retinal disparity. Anyone with two normal eyes can readily be convinced of this fact by fixating binocularly an object point and then displacing one eye slightly by pressure from a finger. The object point, which appeared single before pressure was applied to the globe, is now seen in diplopia because it is no longer imaged on corresponding retinal areas.

16.2.2.2 Motor fusion

The term motor fusion refers to the ability to align the eyes in such a manner that sensory fusion can be maintained. The stimulus for these fusional eye movements is retinal disparity outside *Panum's area* and the two eyes are moving in opposite directions. Unlike sensory fusion, which occurs between corresponding retinal elements in the fovea and the retinal periphery, motor fusion is the exclusive function of the extrafoveal retinal periphery. No stimulus for motor fusion exists when the images of a fixated visual object fall on the fovea of each eye.

16.2.3 Stereopsis

Convergence is the innervation of the eyes needed to form a moving and sensory image of an object. The activity can also determine the distance between the object and the body, but it is not an effective sense of depth. Under specific circumstances, the combination can affect the judgment of the distance, thus affecting the judgment of the size of the object. For example, when two eyes look at an object at a fixed distance, place a bottom facing prism in front of both eyes. With the increase of the degree of the prism, the two eyes maintain single vision. As the syncretism increases, the object looks smaller and closer. The bottom inward prism object looks bigger and farther. This phenomenon is commonly used in clinical measurement of visual function convergence and divergence, which is called "small out large in".

Visual stereo vision is the strongest depth cue. Depth cue is subconscious and can be formed naturally without conscious feeling. When two eyes look at an object, the object image is formed on the corresponding points of the retinas of the two eyes, while the object image of the other eye is in a slightly different position, that is, it is not on the monocular circle, but the object image is formed on the corresponding points of the retinas of the two eyes, it is still in the Panum's area. At this time, the two eyes can still fuse. The amount of deviation between the fixation point and non-fixation point is called horizontal *bilocular disparity*, which can make the visual system produce stereo vision.

16.2.3.1 Stereoscopic acuity

The responsiveness to disparate stimulations has its limits. There is a minimal disparity beyond which no stereoscopic effect is produced. This limiting disparity characterizes a person's stereoscopic acuity.

Stereoscopic acuity depends on many factors and is influenced greatly by the method used in determining it. In refined laboratory examinations and with highly trained subjects, stereoscopic acuities as low as 2 to 7 seconds of arc have been found. There are no standardized clinical stereoscopic acuity tests comparable to visual acuity tests, and no results of mass examinations. Generally speaking, a threshold of 15 to 30 seconds obtained in clinical tests may be regarded as excellent.

Visual acuity has some relation to stereoscopic acuity. Stereoscopic acuity cannot be greater than the vernier acuity of the stimulated retinal area. Stereoscopic acuity decreases, as does visual acuity, from the center to the periphery of the retina. However, despite this relationship, stereopsis is a function not linearly correlated with visual acuity. It has been shown, for instance, that reduction of visual acuity with neutral filters over one eye does not raise the stereoscopic threshold, even if the acuity is lowered to as low as 0.3. A further decrease in vision to 0.2 greatly increases the threshold and with a decrease in acuity of the covered eye to 0.1, stereopsis is absent. On the other hand, spectacle blur decreases stereo acuity more than ordinary visual acuity. This observation raises doubts about the value of stereo acuity testing being advocated by many as a foolproof visual screening method for preschool children.

Since there is a stereoscopic threshold, it follows that stereopsis cannot work beyond a certain critical distance.

16.2.3.2 Stereopsis and fusion

Although it is true that sensory fusion is essential for the highest degree of stereopsis, lower degrees of stereopsis may occur in the absence of sensory fusion and even in the presence of heterotropia. Examples are microtropia and small angle esotropia. Moreover, it has been shown experimentally that binocular depth discrimination may occur with diplopia. For instance, if a peripherally seen wire is located to the left and at some distance in front of a binocularly fixated wire, as in a horopter apparatus, the peripheral wire appears in (physiologic) diplopia. One can attempt to place a second peripheral wire, located in the right half of the field, in line with the left peripheral wire. The closer the left peripheral wire is to the centrally fixated wire, the more accurate is the setting of the wire on the right. The accuracy decreases with increasing distance from the central wire, and eventually, the settings are made by pure chance, indicating that the wire on the right is no longer placed by the criterion of stereopsis, and stereopsis has broken down. These observations are important for the theory of stereopsis. Whereas this experiment shows that sensory fusion of disparate retinal images is not essential for binocular depth discrimination, it must be emphasized that to obtain higher degrees of stereopsis the similar parts of a *stereogram* must be fused to obtain a frame of reference.

On the other hand, sensory fusion (i.e., the ability to unify images falling on corresponding retinal areas) does not keep the presence of stereopsis. There are patients who readily fuse similar targets and who may have normal fusional amplitudes but who have no stereopsis. Such patients suppress selectively the disparately imaged elements of a stereogram seen by one eye.

16.3 ABNORMALITIES OF BINOCULAR VISION

There are many factors in the non-strabismus binocular visual abnormalities, mainly regulation and accumulation and dispersion factors, or single factor, or multiple factors. In general, with normal accommodation and vergence, we can maintain the normal binocular vision. The relationship among accommodation, vergence and pupil contraction is called the *triad* which means accommodation, vergence and contracting of the pupil increase simultaneously. Its advantage is increasing the efficiency and *synchronization* of *innervation*.

There are 12 common basic non-strabismus abnormal binocular vision:
- Divergence excess
- Divergence insufficiency
- Convergence excess
- Convergence insufficiency
- Basic exophoria
- Basic esophoria
- Accommodative insufficiency
- Accommodative excess
- Accommodative infacility
- Ill-sustained accommodation
- Aniseikonia
- Fusional vergence disorder (FVD)

Abnormalities of binocular vision include suppression, amblyopia, confusion, diplopia, etc.

16.3.1 Suppression

The interaction of competition and suppression between binocular images is a pervasive aspect of binocular vision. When the relative differences between the two eyes' images become too large, they compete for awareness and the brain must adopt a strategy to prevent the unwanted consequences of confusion and diplopia. One possible solution is to alternate visual awareness between the two images (binocular rivalry), but another strategy is to simply suppress one image (inter-ocular suppression), so that the other one dominates perception. In other words, inter-ocular suppression arises when the two eyes are stimulated with incompatible images and amblyopia is subsequently induced.

16.3.2 Amblyopia

Amblyopia is a disorder of the visual system characterized by decrease in the best corrected visual acuity in one or both eyes with no ocular pathology. Common amblyopia risk factors include *anisometropic* or high refractive error, strabismus, cataract, and *ptosis*. Often a conservative approach with spectacles is enough to prevent amblyopia.

16.3.3 Confusion

It occurs due to formation of image of two different objects on the corresponding points of two retina and it has not enough power to superimpose two different images to form one complete image.

16.3.4 Diplopia

16.3.4.1 Binocular diplopia

The same object projects onto the non-corresponding points of the retinas of both eyes, that is, one is onto the fovea of the fixation eye and other is onto the peripheral retinas, so the same object is perceived as two objects.

16.3.4.2 Uniocular diplopia

Uniocular diplopia refers to the appearance of an object in double from the affected eye even when the normal eye is closed. It may affect just one eye or both eyes. Common causes of uniocular diplopia are as follows: *subluxated lens*, double pupil, *incipient cataract*, keratoconus, eccentric IOL.

Chapter 17
Common Clinical Conversations

EYE EXAM
MYOPIA
GLAUCOMA
CATARACT
RETINAL DETACHMENT
IRIDOCYCLITIS
CONJUNCTIVITIS
OPTOMETRY AND OPTOMETRIST
REFRACTIVE ERROR
STEP BY STEP PROCEDURES OF SUBJECTIVE REFRACTION

17.1 EYE EXAM (DIALOGUE BETWEEN A REPORTER AND A DOCTER)

Q: Hi, Peter. Do you think everyone needs to have an eye exam?

A: Sure! It is advisable to have an eye exam every year. An eye exam helps detect eye problems at their earliest stage — when they're most treatable. Regular eye exams can give your eye care professional the chance to help you correct or adapt to vision changes. They can also provide advice on eye protection and give clues to your overall health.

Q: Do people of all ages receive the same type of eye exam?

A: Not necessarily. The eye exam can vary depending on the age group. The frequency of eye exams can be determined by several factors, such as your age, health status, and the risk of developing eye problems. General guidelines are as follows:

- *For children 3 years and younger*: Your child's pediatrician will likely check your child's eyes for healthy eye development and look for the most common childhood eye problems —amblyopia (*Figure 17-1a*), cross-eyes, or misaligned eyes (*Figure 17-1b*). A more comprehensive eye exam between the ages of 3 and 5 will look for problems with vision and eye alignment.

- *For school-age children and adolescents*: Have your child's vision checked before he or she enters kindergarten. Your child's doctor can recommend how frequent eye exams should be after that.
- *For adults*: In general, if you are healthy and you have no symptoms of vision problems, the American Academy of Ophthalmology(AAO) recommends having a complete eye exam at age 40, when some vision changes and eye diseases are likely to start. Based on the results of your screening, your eye doctor can recommend how often you should have future eye exams. If you're 60 or older, have your eyes checked every year or two. Have your eyes checked more often if you: a. wear glasses (*Figure 17-2a*) or contact lenses (*Figure 17-2b*); b. have a family history of eye disease or loss of vision; c. have a chronic disease that puts you at greater risk of eye disease, such as diabetes (*Figure 17-3*), high blood pressure (*Figure 17-4*), high cholesterol; d. take medications that have serious eye side effects.

Q: Sure! Thank you so much!

17.2 MYOPIA (DIALOGUE BETWEEN A REPORTER AND A DOCTER)

Q: Hi, Peter. I'm sorry to bother you. Could you please tell me what myopia means?

A: OK. At first, your eye has two parts that focus images: The cornea is the clear, dome-shaped front surface of your eye. The lens is a clear structure about the size and shape of an M&M's candy. Then, in order for you to see, light has to pass through the cornea and lens. They bend (refract) the light, so that the light is focused directly on the nerve tissues (actually the retina) at the back of your eye. These tissues translate light into signals sent to the brain, which enables you to perceive images. That's normal condition (*Figure 17-5a*). However, many people have refractive errors. Nearsightedness is a refractive error. This problem occurs when the shape or condition of the cornea — or the shape of the eye itself — results in an inaccurate focusing of the light passing into the eye. Nearsightedness usually results from the eye being too long or oval-shaped rather than round. It may also result from the curve of the cornea being too steep. These changes result in light rays coming to a point in front of the retina and crossing. The messages sent from the retina to the brain are perceived as blurry (*Figure 17-5b*).

Q: Wow, what are the risk factors of myopia?

A: Myopia is thought to be caused by a combination of genetic and environmental factors. Obviously, the ill habits of using eyes, such as short outdoor time, reading for a long time, reading too close and other acquired factors are the main reasons for the rising trend of myopia. Of course, the hereditary factor gets an important position in myopia, too. Over the last two decades, more than 400 associated gene loci have been mapped for myopia and refractive errors via family linkage analyses, candidate gene studies, genome-wide association studies (GWAS), and next-generation sequencing (NGS).

Q: What can we do for myopia control?

A: Many ways are beneficial for myopia control. Let me show you the most effective three ways.

- No.1 is the sufficient outdoor activity(*Figure 17-6a*). Students should keep outdoor activity 2 hours every day at least. You can play tennis, or play basketball, no matter what, just to enjoy the sunshine.
- No.2 is orthokeratology (*Figure 17-6b*). It's a good way for most children to control myopia, but it's not suitable for everyone. Remember, people who wear contact lenses must go to the hospital regularly for review.
- No.3 is the 0.01% atropine eye drops (*Figure 17-6c*). It has been shown by research that low dose atropine eye drops can be used for myopia control. After comparing many concentrations, 0.01% was found to be the most suitable concentration.

Q: So, what other approaches can we use to get the same effect?

A: Ummm, there are many types of glasses we can choose from. We can recommend peripheral defocus spectacle glasses (*Figure 17-7a*) for patients who don't like contact lenses, or we can recommend soft defocus contact lenses for patients who pursue the comfort (*Figure 17-7b*). However, we can't guarantee that each type of glasses will work equally well in myopia control.

Q: OK, it sounds a little complicated. I want to know how to choose the best way.

A: It depends. Prescribing the orthokeratology lenses, atropine eye drops, and peripheral defocus spectacle glasses need a comprehensive eye examination, including eye pressure, ocular surface, axial length, keratometric power, refraction, binocular vision, and so on. After that, everyone can choose the best way for them with our advice.

Q: Is there any advice for people without myopia?

A: If you want to prevent the occurrence of myopia, please remember do eye examinations regularly. In daily life, No.1 is spend more time outside; No.2 is reduce the amount of time you spend reading or looking at screens; No.3 is adjust your computer's screen settings; No.4 is avoid reading in dimly lit rooms; No.5 is eat healthy foods that help preserve eyesight.

Q: You've really helped us a lot! Thank you so much!

17.3 GLAUCOMA (DIALOGUE BETWEEN A REPORTER AND A DOCTER)

Q: Hi, Peter. How can I know if a person has glaucoma?

A: Ummm, It's a good question. The first thing is to know what glaucoma actually is, and we should know how to differentiate other similar conditions with glaucoma, such as intraocular hypertension. And we should differentiate all kinds of glaucoma, like normal-tension glaucoma, primary open-angle glaucoma, primary angle-closure glaucoma, etc. To diagnose it, we should find some evidence in the eye, including the eye pressure (*Figure 17-8a*) and the C/D ratio(*Figure 17-8b*). In addition, visual field tests(*Figure 17-8c*), visual acuity tests, and fundus examinations are essential.

Q: So, what is glaucoma?

A: Glaucoma is the leading cause of irreversible blindness. Glaucoma is a group of eye diseases that can cause vision loss and blindness by damaging a nerve in the back of your eye called the optic nerve. The symptoms can start so slowly that you may not notice them. The only way to find out if you have glaucoma is to get a comprehensive dilated eye exam. There's no cure for glaucoma, but early treatment can often stop the damage and protect your vision. Eye pressure is the only known modifiable risk factor for glaucoma and is the target of current treatment regimens. Treatments include prescription eye drops, oral medicines, laser therapy, surgery, or a combination of methods.

Q: Who is at risk for glaucoma?

A: Anyone can get glaucoma, but some people are at higher risk. The risk is higher if you are older than 60, if you have a family history of glaucoma, especially a sibling relationship, if your corneas are thin in the center, if you have extreme nearsightedness or farsightedness, and if you take corticosteroid medicines, especially eye drops, for a long time.

Q: What should patients at risk for glaucoma do first?

A: Patients should proactively talk to their doctors about their glaucoma risk and ask how often they need to get tested. If someone is at high risk, he needs a comprehensive eye exam every one to two years. Regular comprehensive eye exams can help detect glaucoma in its early stages, before significant damage occurs. In addition, serious eye injuries can lead to glaucoma. Wear eye protection when using power tools or playing sports.

Q: What are the symptoms of glaucoma patients?

A: Most people with glaucoma do not notice symptoms until they begin to lose eyesight. As glaucoma damages optic nerve fibers(*Figure 17-9*), small blind spots may begin to develop. These spots usually occur on the side or in the peripheral vision. Many people do not notice the blind spots until significant optic nerve damage has already happened. Blindness can result when the entire nerve is destroyed. One type of angle-closure glaucoma, called acute angle-closure glaucoma, does produce noticeable symptoms. This is because there is a quick buildup of pressure in the eye. Each person may experience symptoms differently, which include blurred or narrowed field of vision, severe pain in the eyes, seeing halos or "rainbows" around lights, nausea, vomiting, and headache. The symptoms of acute angle-closure glaucoma may resemble those of other eye problems. Receiving medical attention quickly when first noticing symptoms can help prevent blindness.

Q: What is the latest research on glaucoma?

A: As we all know, glaucoma is known as the "silent blinder" because there are no noticeable symptoms in the early stages, early detection and treatment for glaucoma are the most important steps to prevent vision loss. Scientists are focusing on what causes glaucoma and how to find it earlier and treat it better.

Q: wow, that's great, thank you!

17.4 CATARACT (DIALOGUE BETWEEN A REPORTER AND A DOCTER)

Q: Hi, Peter. I see many old people with white pupils. What is that?

A: That's cataract. A cataract is a cloudy area in the lens of your eye. Cataracts are very common as you get older. In fact, more than half of all people age 80 or older either have cataracts or have had surgery to get rid of cataracts. At first, you may not notice that you have a cataract. But over time, cataracts can make your vision blurry, hazy, or less colorful. You may have trouble reading or doing other everyday activities. The good news is that surgery can get rid of cataracts. Cataract surgery is safe and can correct vision problems caused by cataracts (*Figure 17-10*).

Q: What causes cataract?

A: Aging is the most common cause. This is due to normal eye changes that begin to happen after age 40. That is when normal proteins in the lens start to break down. This is what causes the lens to get cloudy. People over age 60 usually start to have some clouding of their lenses. However, vision problems may not happen until years later. Most age-related cataracts develop gradually. Other cataracts can develop more quickly, such as those in younger people or those in people with diabetes. Doctors cannot predict how quickly a person's cataract will develop.

Q: How do I know if I am at risk for cataracts?

A: Your risk for cataracts goes up as you get older. You're also at higher risk if you:
- Have certain health problems, like diabetes.
- Smoke.
- Drink too much alcohol.
- Have a family history of cataracts.
- Have had an eye injury, eye surgery, or radiation treatment on your upper body.
- Have spent a lot of time in the sun.
- Take steroids (medicines used to treat a variety of health problems, like arthritis and rashes).

If you're worried you might be at risk for cataracts, talk with your doctor. Ask if there is anything you can do to lower your risk.

Q: Wow, thank you. So, is there any medicine or vision therapy for cataract?

A: No, we usually suggest patients do surgery for cataracts. However, we should take notice that cataracts can cause amblyopia if it happens to newborns (*Figure 17-11a*), and it's best to remove the cataract as soon as possible, then we need to prescribe contact lenses or spectacle glasses for the baby (*Figure 17-11b*). IOL surgery is also suggested sometimes. For amblyopia caused by congenital cataract, we can do some vision therapy after cataract surgery. The goal is to improve vision.

Q: Cataracts are terrible. How can we prevent them?

A: People can take steps to protect their eyes and delay cataracts.

- Wear sunglasses and a hat with a brim to block the sun.
- Quit smoking.
- Eat healthy. Eat plenty of fruits and vegetables — especially dark, leafy greens like spinach, kale, and collard greens.
- Get a dilated eye exam every year.

Q: Once I have a cataract diagnosis, what should I do?

A: Have an eye exam every year if you're older than 65, or every two years if younger. Get the right eyeglasses or contact lenses to correct your vision. When it becomes difficult to complete your regular activities, consider cataract surgery.

Q: How does cataract surgery work?

A: During cataract surgery, your eye surgeon will remove your eye's cloudy natural lens. Then he or she will replace it with an artificial lens. This new lens is called an intraocular lens (or IOL). However, people who have had cataract surgery may have their vision become hazy again years later. This is usually because the lens capsule has become cloudy. The capsule is the part of your eye that holds the IOL in place. Fortunately, your ophthalmologist can use a laser to open the cloudy capsule and restore clear vision. This is called a capsulotomy. Cataracts are a very common reason people lose vision, but they can be treated.

Q: I see. Thank you so much!

17.5 RETINAL DETACHMENT (DIALOGUE BETWEEN A REPORTER AND A DOCTER)

Q: Hi, Peter. What is retinal detachment? I heard people say it can cause blindness?

A: Sure! Retinal detachment is an eye problem that happens when your retina (a light-sensitive layer of tissue in the back of your eye) is pulled away from its normal position at the back of your eye.

Q: What causes retinal detachment?

A: There are many causes of retinal detachment, but the most common causes are aging or eye injury. There are 2 types (*Figure 17-12*) of retinal detachment: rhegmatogenous and non-rhegmatogenous (tractional or exudative). Each type happens because of a different problem that causes your retina to move away from the back of your eye.

Q: What are the symptoms of retinal detachment?

A: If only a small part of your retina has detached, you may not have any symptoms. But if more of your retina is detached, you may not be able to see as clearly as normal, and you may notice other sudden symptoms, including:

- A lot of new floaters (small dark spots or squiggly lines that float across your vision) (*Figure 17-13a*).
- Flashes of light in one eye or both eyes.
- A dark shadow or "curtain" on the sides or in the middle of your field of vision(*Figure 17-13b*).

Remember, Retinal detachment is a medical emergency. If you have symptoms of a detached retina, it's important to go to your eye doctor or the emergency room right away. The symptoms of retinal detachment often come on quickly. If the retinal detachment isn't treated right away, more of the retina can detach — which increases the risk of permanent vision loss or blindness.

Q: It's so terrible. Who is at risk for retinal detachment?

A: Anyone can have retinal detachment, but some people are at higher risk. You are at higher risk if:

- You or a family member has had a retinal detachment before.
- You've had a serious eye injury.
- You've had eye surgery, like surgery to treat cataracts.

Some other problems with your eyes may also put you at higher risk, including:

- Diabetic retinopathy (a condition in people with diabetes that affects blood vessels in the retina) (*Figure 17-14a*).
- Extreme nearsightedness, especially a severe type called degenerative myopia.
- Posterior vitreous detachment (when the gel-like fluid in the center of the eye pulls away from the retina) (*Figure 17-14b*).
- Certain other eye diseases, including retinoschisis (*Figure 17-14c*) (when the retina separates into 2 layers) or lattice degeneration (thinning of the retina) (*Figure 17-14d*).

So, talk to your eye doctor if you are concerned about the risk of retinal detachment.

Q: Yeah, I remember you suggested that we should have an eye exam every year, so how can we prevent retinal detachment in our life?

A: Since retinal detachment is often caused by aging, there's often no way to prevent it. But you can lower your risk of retinal detachment from an eye injury by wearing safety goggles or other protective eye gear when doing risky activities, like playing sports. If you experience any symptoms of retinal detachment, go to your eye doctor or the emergency room right away. Early treatment can help prevent permanent vision loss.

It's also important to get comprehensive dilated eye exams regularly. A dilated eye exam can help your eye doctor find a small retinal tear or detachment early before it starts to affect your vision.

Q: Wow, that's great! What should we do if retinal detachment happens?

A: If treatment of a detached retina is not performed immediately (within approximately 24 hours), permanent partial or complete vision loss can result. Retinal detachment surgery is considered an emergency procedure. The goal of surgery is to reattach the retina to the back of the eye as soon as possible so that the blood supply can be reestablished. Several different procedures can be performed to repair a detached retina; the type of surgery will depend on how severe the detachment is, and which area of the eye is involved in the retinal detachment. In some circumstances, a person will require more than one type of surgery to effectively repair the retina.

Q: It's amazing! Is there any new technique for the retina?

A: Yeah, there is no end to science. We all know that the human visual system enables perceiving, learning, remembering, and recognizing elementary visual information (light, colors, and images), which has inspired the development of biomimicry visual system-based electronic devices. Proof-of-concept devices, by simplifying the circuitry and providing dual-mode functions, can contribute significantly to the development of bionics design and broaden the horizon for smart artificial retinas in the human visual system. In the future, if a patient develops retinal detachment, we hope that the artificial retina will become the last option after surgery fails.

Q: wow, that's wonderful! Thank you so much!

17.6 IRIDOCYCLITIS (DIALOGUE BETWEEN A REPORTER AND A DOCTER)

Q: Hi, Peter. I recently heard of a new disease called iridocyclitis. I've never heard of this before. What is it?

A: Eyes are one of the most sensitive organs in the body and tend to get easily irritated due to several different reasons. Iridocyclitis is an eye condition where the iris (the colored part of the eye) and the ciliary body (the muscles and tissues that are involved in focusing the eye) are inflamed(*Figure 17-15*). The iris is the part that lends a specific color to the eye. Therefore, whenever you see blue-grey, green, brown or black eyes, it is the iris that you are seeing. The iris controls the amount of light entering the eye through the pupil, which is the dark opening at the center of the eye. Right next to the iris is the ciliary body, which is a ring of tissue that encircles the lens of the eye. The ciliary body helps to control the shape of the lens and secretes aqueous humor, a fluid which provides nutrients to the eye.

Q: What are the causes of iridocyclitis?

A: It may also be called iritis or anterior uveitis. The causes of iridocyclitis are diverse, may be endogenous or exogenous. Any condition that causes damage or inflammation to the iris or ciliary body can cause iridocyclitis. Often, iridocyclitis develops due to traumatic damage to the eye (wounds, contusions, ophthalmic operations) or inflammation of the iris (keratitis). Iridocyclitis can be caused by transferred viral, bacterial or protozoal diseases (influenza, measles, HSV, staphylococcal and streptococcal infections, tuberculosis, gonorrhea, chlamydia, toxoplasmosis, malaria, etc.), as well as existing foci of chronic infection in the nasopharynx and oral cavity (sinusitis, tonsillitis). The cause of iridocyclitis may be rheumatoid conditions (rheumatism, Still's disease, autoimmune thyroiditis, Bechterev's disease, Reiter and Sjogren syndromes), metabolic disorders (gout, diabetes), systemic diseases of unknown etiology (sarcoidosis, Behcet's disease, Vogt-Koyanagi-Harada syndrome). The prevalence of iridocyclitis among patients with rheumatic and infectious diseases is about 40% of cases. Sometimes no apparent reason for the iridocyclitis is found.

Q: What are the symptoms of iridocyclitis?

A: The severity and characteristics of the course of iridocyclitis depend on the nature and duration of exposure to the antigen, the level of permeability of the hematophthalmic barrier, genotype and immune status of the organism. Symptoms generally include blurred vision, eye pain, sensitivity to light, red eyes, and rarely vision loss. With iridocyclitis, unilateral eye damage is usually observed. The first signs of acute iridocyclitis are general redness and pain in the eye, with a characteristic significant increase in pain when pressing on the eyeball. Patients with iridocyclitis have photophobia, lacrimation, a slight decrease in visual acuity (within 2~3 lines), and the appearance of a "fog" in front of their eyes. The course of iridocyclitis is characterized by a noticeable change in the color of the inflamed iris (greenish or rusty-red) and a decrease in the clarity of its pattern. Different types of iridocyclitis have their own clinical features.

Q: How is iridocyclitis diagnosed?

A: The diagnosis of iridocyclitis is established by the results of a comprehensive examination: ophthalmological, laboratory diagnostic, radiological, consulting of the patient by narrow specialists. Differential diagnosis of iridocyclitis and other diseases accompanied by swelling and redness of the eyes, such as acute conjunctivitis, keratitis, acute attack of primary glaucoma, is carried out. Iridocyclitis can be classified as:

- *Acute iridocyclitis*: Sudden onset, with a usual duration of 3 weeks although may last up to 6 weeks. It does not take very long for acute iridocyclitis to recede.
- *Chronic iridocyclitis*: Chronic iridocyclitis has a much slower onset as compared to the acute iridocyclitis. It also has a more prolonged existence and lasts for more than three months.
- *Recurrent iridocyclitis*: This is one of the most common types of iridocyclitis and keeps on coming back even after recovery. With this type of iridocyclitis, relapsing is quite a common occurrence.

Q: How is iridocyclitis treated?

A: Treatment of iridocyclitis should be timely and, if possible, aimed at eliminating the cause of its occurrence. Most cases of iridocyclitis clear up by themselves within a few days. If iridocyclitis is caused by an infection or a specific condition, then treating this underlying cause will usually relieve the symptoms. Treatment should be started early to minimize vision damage. Treatments may include corticosteroids (these may be oral, topical, periocular, intraocular, or intravenous). Iridocyclitis is associated with a favorable prognosis. If the patient is given proper treatment, a complete recovery is possible without any complications during the process. However, the condition has high chances of relapsing even after a complete healing. If it is not properly treated in the ensuing period, it can lead to a very poor prognosis.

Q: Sounds like a tough disease to deal with! Thank you so much!

17.7 CONJUNCTIVITIS (DIALOGUE BETWEEN A REPORTER AND A DOCTER)

Q: Hi, Peter. My wife said she was diagnosed with pink eye. What's that?

A: Oh, pink eye refers to conjunctivitis.

Q: So, it's the inflammation of conjunctiva?

A: Yes, you are right. Pink eye (conjunctivitis) is an inflammation or infection of the transparent membrane (conjunctiva) that lines your eyelid and covers the white part of your eyeball(*Figure 17-16*). When small blood vessels in the conjunctiva become inflamed, they're more visible. This is what causes the whites of your eyes to appear reddish or pink. Pink eye is commonly caused by a bacterial or viral infection, an allergic reaction, or — in babies — an incompletely opened tear duct.

Q: How can I prevent it? How do I keep my wife from infecting me?

A: Practice good hygiene to control the spread of pink eye. For instance:
- Don't touch your eyes with your hands.
- Wash your hands often.
- Use a clean towel and washcloth daily.
- Don't share towels or washcloths.
- Change your pillowcases often.
- Throw away your eye cosmetics, such as mascara.
- Don't share eye cosmetics or personal eye-care items.

Q: Thank you. I get it! Just keep distance from my wife recently. How are the different types of conjunctivitis treated? What can I do for my wife?

A: There are times when it is important to seek medical care for conjunctivitis (pink eye). However, this is not always necessary. To help relieve some of the inflammation and dryness caused by conjunctivitis, she can use cold compresses and artificial tears. Your wife should also stop wearing contact lenses until her eye doctor says it's okay to start wearing them again. If she did not need to see a doctor, do not wear her contacts until she no longer has symptoms of pink eye. She should see a healthcare provider if she has conjunctivitis along with any of the following:
- Pain in the eye(s).

- Sensitivity to light or blurred vision that does not improve when discharge is wiped from the eye(s).
- Intense redness in the eye(s).
- Symptoms that get worse or don't improve, including pink eye thought to be caused by bacteria which does not improve after 24 hours of antibiotic use.
- A weakened immune system, for example from HIV infection, cancer treatment, or other medical conditions or treatments.
- Keep in mind that newborns with symptoms of conjunctivitis should be seen by a doctor right away.

Q: Sure! I heard conjunctivitis is contagious and people can't go to work while they are sick.

A: Several viruses and bacteria can cause conjunctivitis (pink eye), some of which are very contagious. Each of these types of germs can spread from person to person in different ways. They usually spread from an infected person to others through close personal contact, such as touching or shaking hands, the air by coughing and sneezing, touching an object or surface with germs on it, then touching your eyes before washing your hands. So, if your wife has conjunctivitis but do not has fever or other symptoms, she may be allowed to remain at work or school with her doctor's approval. However, if she still has symptoms, and her activities at work or school include close contact with other people, she should not attend.

Q: Thank you so much!

17.8 OPTOMETRY AND OPTOMETRIST (DIALOGUE BETWEEN A REPORTER AND A DOCTER)

Q: Hi, Peter. I know you are an optometrist, so what is the definition of optometrist?

A: If you love people, want to improve their lives, and are scientifically minded, a career as an optometrist is waiting for you! As one of the five senses, sight is hugely important—and in a modern world filled with computer screens and mobile phone screens, it is increasingly necessary for everyone to have access to specialist eye care and attend regular eye check-ups. As an optometrist, you'll be trained to examine the eye, to detect and diagnose any abnormalities and diseases, and to prescribe glasses or contact lenses. Studying optometry can lead you to an exciting and varied career. You'll get to put your knowledge into practice with diverse placement opportunities, and will learn about the issues that can affect eyesight. This may lead you on to further study, with options to specialise and gain further qualifications in areas such as glaucoma, contact lens prescribing, and low vision. The health-care profession concerned especially with examining the eye for defects and faults of refraction, with prescribing correctional lenses or eye exercises, with diagnosing diseases of the eye, and with treating such diseases or referring them for treatment.

Q: What is the difference between an optometrist and an ophthalmologist?

A: An optometrist is trained to examine the eyes and test vision. They can also prescribe spectacles or lenses. Whereas ophthalmologists are surgical and medical specialists who perform operations on eyes.

Q: Why study optometry at university?

A: There are many issues that can affect the eyes including blindness, cataracts, and glaucoma, and by studying optometry, you will be at the forefront of change in this pivotal space. You'll receive a professionally recognised qualification that will enable you to practice as an optometrist, and because optometry is an occupational degree, it is highly likely you will find employment soon after graduating. You'll examine patients' eyes, give advice, prescribe and fit spectacles, and ultimately, you'll be able to make a huge difference to peoples' lives. So, if you're the sort of person who loves science and learning the intricacies of how something works, and who also has a passion for working with people and seeing results of their study in real life situations, then optometry might just be the course for you! You will also develop transferable skills in communication, problem-solving, and critical evaluation. These will be useful no matter which career path you choose.

Q: What can you do with an optometry degree?

A: Optometry is a growing profession in China. You will need to successfully complete your degree in optometry to become a practising optometrist. Graduates tend to work in hospitals, opticians, or larger retail stores. While many companies run graduate schemes open to those holding a degree in optometry, there are also opportunities to stay in academia through further study. When you are a qualified optometrist, there will be opportunities to study further, or to specialise in an area of optometry, such as glaucoma research.

Q: Wow, it's so good. I like it!

17.9 REFRACTIVE ERROR (DIALOGUE BETWEEN A REPORTER AND A DOCTER)

Q: Hi, peter. My son said he can't see the blackboard clear these days. What's wrong with him?

A: He might need a refraction test to determine if he has any refractive errors. Refractive errors are a type of vision problem that makes it difficult for people to see clearly. These occur when the shape of the eye prevents light from focusing directly on the back of the eye, resulting in blurry vision and other symptoms. While refractive errors are common, many people don't realize that they could be seeing better. This is why regular eye exams are crucial. If you have refractive errors, your eye doctor can prescribe glasses or contact lenses to enhance your vision.

Q: But what causes refractive errors?

A: Refractive errors can be caused by:
- Eyeball length (when the eyeball grows too long or too short).

- Problems with the shape of the cornea (the clear outer layer of the eye).
- A thicker or thinner lens than normal.

Q: Are all the refractive errors the same? What are the types of refractive errors?

A: Absolutely not. There are 3 common types of refractive errors:

- Nearsightedness (myopia) (*Figure 17-17a*) makes far-away objects look blurry. It happens when the eyeball grows too long from front to back, or when there are problems with the shape of the cornea (clear front layer of the eye) or the lens (an inner part of the eye that helps the eye focus). These problems make light focus in front of the retina, instead of on it.
- Farsightedness (hyperopia) (*Figure 17-17b*) makes nearby objects look blurry. It happens when the eyeball grows too short from front to back, or when there are problems with the shape of the cornea or lens. These problems make light focus behind the retina, instead of on it. People with farsightedness are usually born with it.
- Astigmatism(*Figure 17-17c*) can make far away and nearby objects look blurry or distorted. It happens when the cornea or lens has a different shape than normal, which makes light bend differently as it enters the eye. Some people with astigmatism are born with it, but many people develop it as children or young adults. People with astigmatism can also have another refractive error, like nearsightedness or farsightedness.

Q: What are the symptoms of refractive errors?

A: The most common symptom is blurry vision. Other symptoms include:

- Double vision.
- Hazy vision.
- Seeing a glare or halo around bright lights.
- Squinting.
- Headaches.
- Eye strain (when your eyes feel tired or sore).
- Trouble focusing when reading or looking at a screen.

Some people may not notice the symptoms of refractive errors. It's important to get eye exams regularly, so your eye doctor can make sure you're seeing as clearly as possible. If you wear glasses or contact lenses and still have these symptoms, you might need a new prescription. Talk to your eye doctor and get an eye exam if you are having trouble with your vision.

Q: Am I at risk for refractive errors?

A: Anyone can have refractive errors, but you're at higher risk if you have family members who wear glasses or contact lenses. Most types of refractive errors, like nearsightedness, usually start in childhood. Talk with your doctor about your risk for refractive errors, and ask how often you need to get checked. Early diagnosis of refractive errors is particularly essential for children, because a child's academic progress can be affected by poor vision. Also, if a child's refractive errors are not addressed timely, amblyopia might develop. When standard eye charts cannot be used for younger children, their vision may need to be assessed by a retinoscopy — an exam that observes the reflection of light off the retina. This test may require dilation of pupils using eyedrops.

Q: How are refractive errors treated?

A: Treatments for refractive errors include eyeglasses, contact lenses, vision correction surgery such as LASIK and photorefractive keratectomy (PRK) (*Figure 17-18*). Usually, your eye care specialist will prescribe you glasses or contacts before you have vision correction surgery. However, you might be a good candidate for vision correction surgery right away. Talk to your eye care specialist about which treatment will work the best for you. Remember, vision correction surgery is only for adults!

Q: Thank you so much! I'm taking my son to an eye exam right now!

17.10 STEP BY STEP PROCEDURES OF SUBJECTIVE REFRACTION (DIALOGUE BETWEEN A STUDENT AND A PROFESSOR)

Q: Hi, professor, could you please tell me how to do the subjective refraction?

A: Sure! There are many steps. We do the subjective refraction through phoropter.

Step 1 Start with the results of retinoscopy or autorefractor.

Step 2 Then occlud the left eye, and test the right eye. Fog patient to 20/40 with plus lenses (if patient is myope, may not need to fog).

Step 3 Work towards MOST PLUS, LEAST MINUS BCVA(Best corrected visual acuity).

- Say to patient, "I'm going to give you two choices. They may both be a little blurry, but I want you to tell me which is clearer. This is choice one…" Then take away plus lenses or add minus lenses by 0.25 diopter and say "…or choice two?"
- Remember, each 0.25 D should improve visual acuity by one line. Do not over minus patient (make sure letters are clearer, not smaller or darker).
- If visual acuity is improving, continue advancing with 0.25 D until 20/20 is reached.
- If visual acuity is not improving, then stop and check for astigmatism.

Step 4 Refine the cylinder axis.

- Isolate line of letters. Usually, 20/30 or 20/40. Two lines are worse than best VA. Straddle JCC axis between minus cylinder axis on phoropter (45 degrees on either side with red/white dots between axis).
- Ask patient "Which image is clearer…one …" Then flip the JCC and say, "or two". Which ever choice they like, rotate the minus cylinder axis towards the red mark by 15 degrees (called "chasing the red"). Continue chasing red until reversal of direction. Then move to smaller axis increments until reversal again.
- Keep refining until no difference between image one and two or a midpoint between

both. This result will be cylinder axis.

Step 5 Refine the cylinder power.
- Turn JCC to align red dots with axis of minus cylinder in phoropter.
- Again, ask patient "Which one is clearer, choice one…" Then flip JCC and say, "or …choice two?" Remember to note which flip was clearer.
- If the red dots are landing on the axis with the patient's choice, then add −0.50 D minus cylinder and maintain spherical equivalent(SE) by adding +0.25 D spherical lens (always add ½ of the cylinder in the opposing power to keep consistent image retinal distance). Reversely, if they like the white dots, reduce the minus cylinder or add plus cylinder.
- Repeat asking which JCC flip is clearer, until reversal. Continue to add −0.50 D cylinder and +0.25 D spherical lenses if red is chosen or +0.50 D cylinder and −0.25 D spherical lenses if white is chosen.
- Once reversal found, then change minus cylinder by −0.25 D and no need for spherical equivalent.
- When you get to a point where the patient cannot choose between the two options or is vacillating between two-cylinder powers you've reached your endpoint.

Step 6 Refine the sphere power.
- Fog patient to 20/40 with plus lenses to start.
- Work towards MOST PLUS, LEAST MINUS BCVA.

Step 7 Cylinder power search (if spherical).
- Sometimes we start with a prescription that doesn't have a significant astigmatism component. This is where the "cylinder power search" applies.
- The goal of the "cylinder power search" is to detect any significant uncorrected astigmatism power.
- Start by placing minus cylinder axis at 180 degrees and place JCC over with red dots corresponding to axis (like power check).
- Again, ask patient "Which one is clearer, choice one…" Then flip JCC and say "or …choice two?" Remember to note which flip was clearer.
- If they pick red at 180, then place −0.50 minus cylinder and +0.25 D spherical in phoropter and proceed to check power.
- Or if they like red at 90 degrees, then rotate axis of JCC and phoropter to coordinate with 90 degrees and continue with power cylinder check.
- Once power is found, determine axis refinement with JCC.
- Note: If you show your patient cylinder power at 180 and 90 and they do not feel that one is significantly better than the other, turn the JCC axes to 45 and 135 degrees and ask again.
- Verify for power by asking which image is clearer.
- None are chosen, then the patient is spherical and refraction is complete.

- Now spectacle prescription is final for the right eye. Repeat the process for the left eye now.
- Remember to record VA for each eye and both eyes.

Q: How to do binocular balance (duochrome balance) ?(*Figure 17-19*)

A: The steps for binocular balance are as follows:

- Fog with +0.50 DS.
- Isolate 20/40 Snellen line of letters with duochrome filter.
- Put 3 diopters of BD prism on the right eye and 3 diopters of BU prism on the left eye.
- Verify patient sees two R/G images (right eye sees upper and left eye sees lower).
- If the patient sees only one image, prism needs to be increased.
- Instruct patient to look at the top letters. Ask, "Which side is clearer, the red or the green?" Change spherical lenses of the right eye(0.25 D/step) until equal on red and green sides.
- Instruct patient to look at the lower letters. Ask, "Which side is clearer, the red or the green?" Change spherical lenses of the left eye(0.25 D/step) until equal on red and green sides.
- Once each eye is equal, then ask, "Which is clearer? The top or bottom image?"
- Add plus on the eye which sees the clearer image. If the clarity of both eyes is the same, stop. Check the visual acuity of both eyes at endpoint without prisms.
- If VA is worse than MPMVA, then un-fog to MPMVA.
- If 20/20, add more plus until VA is reduced, then un-fog to MPMVA.
- Of course, You can leave the dominant eye seeing clearer sometimes.

Q: I get it! thank you!

Appendix

Chapter 2
Anatomy and Physiology of the Eye

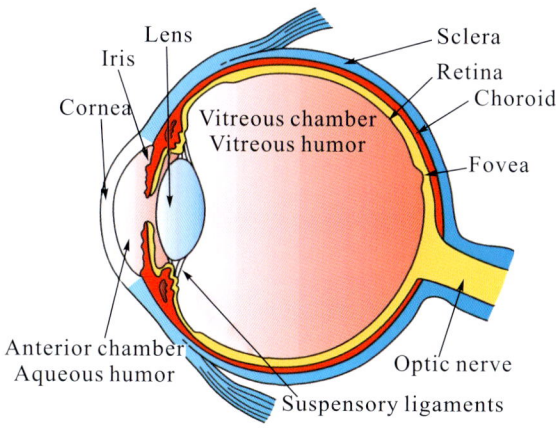

Figure 2-1 Gross anatomy of the eyeball

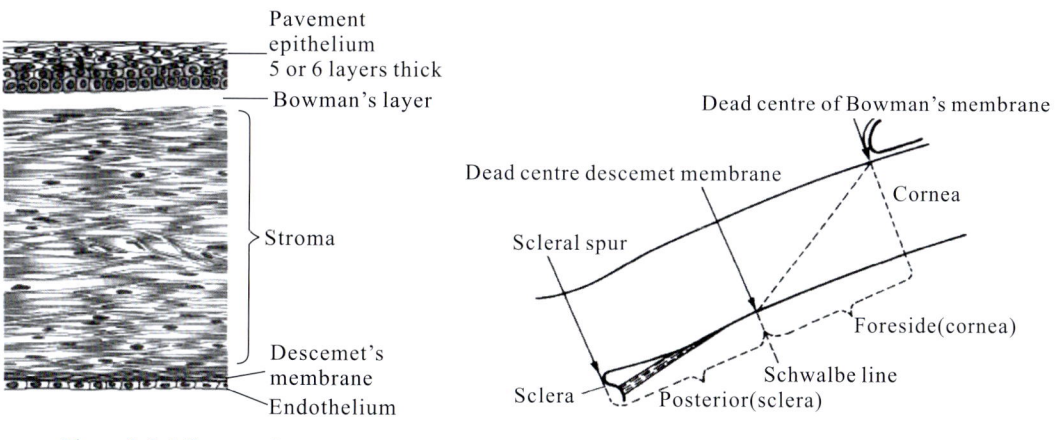

Figure 2-2 Microscopic structure of the cornea

Figure 2-3 Limbus

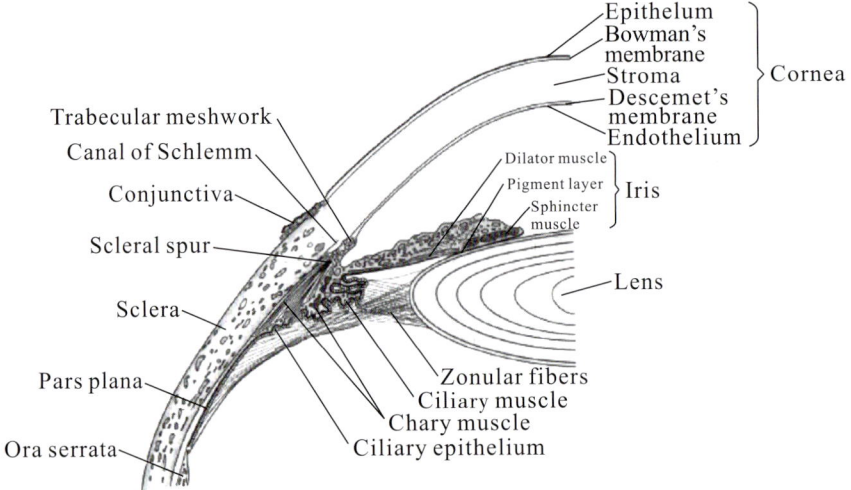

Figure 2-4 Anterior section of the eyeball

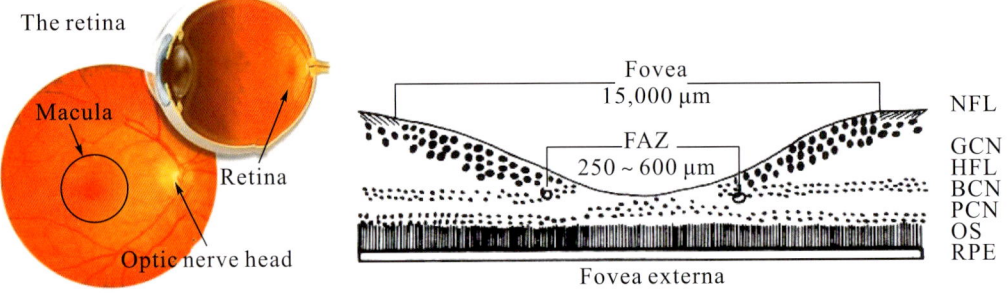

Figure 2-5 Retina

Figure 2-6 Fovea externa

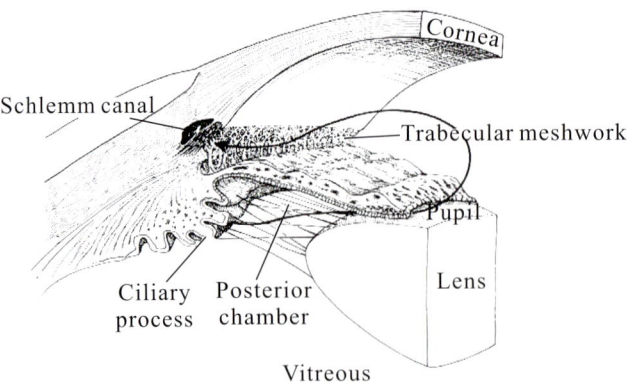

Figure 2-7 The channel for aqueous humor

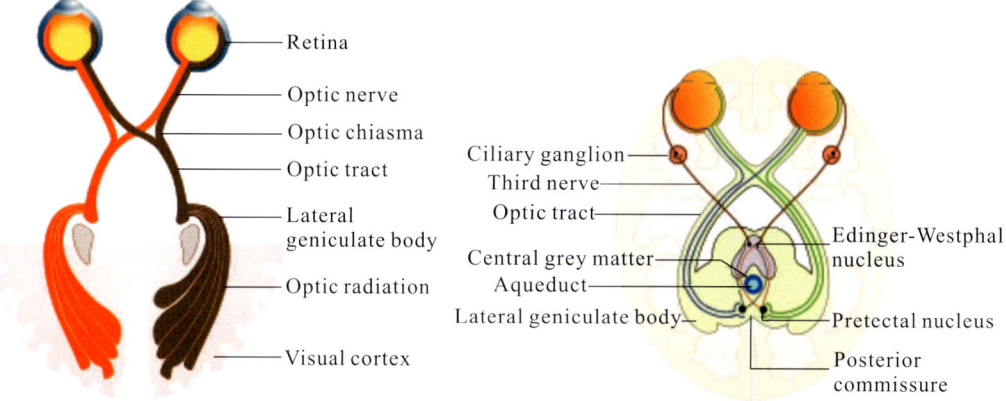

Figure 2-8 Anatomy of the visual pathway

Figure 2-9 Pathway of the light reflex

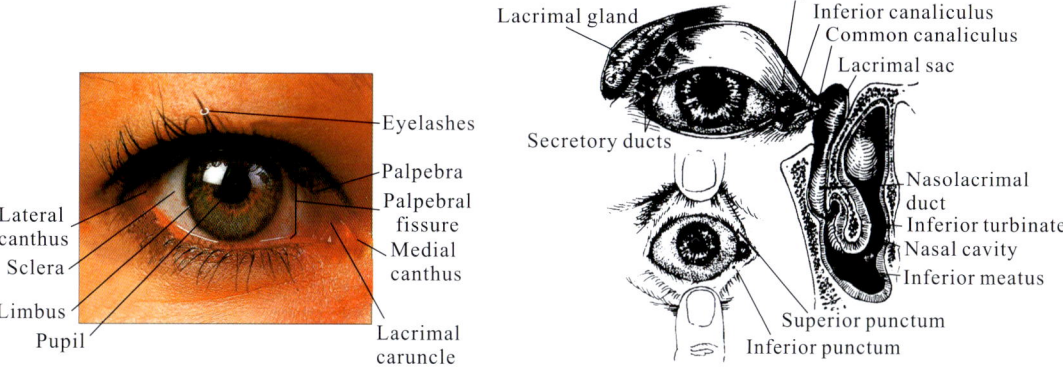

Figure 2-10 Eyelids

Figure 2-11 Lacrimal apparatus

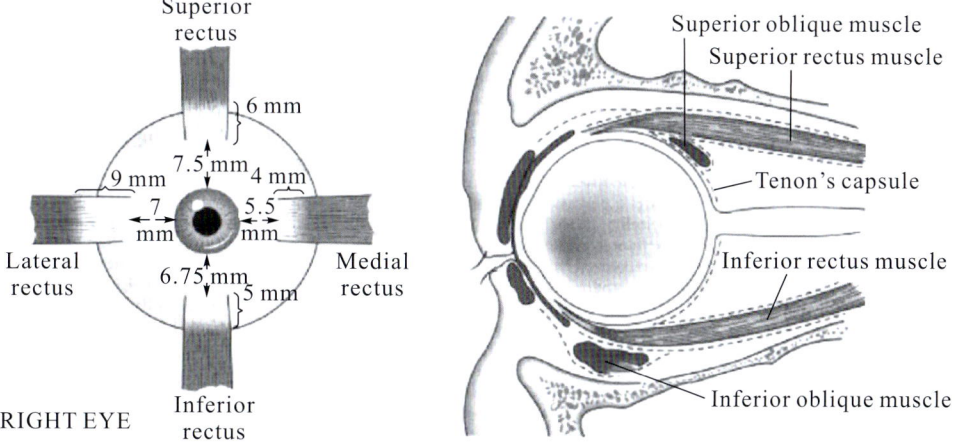

Figure 2-12 Extraocular muscles

Chapter 3
Clinic Methods in Optometry

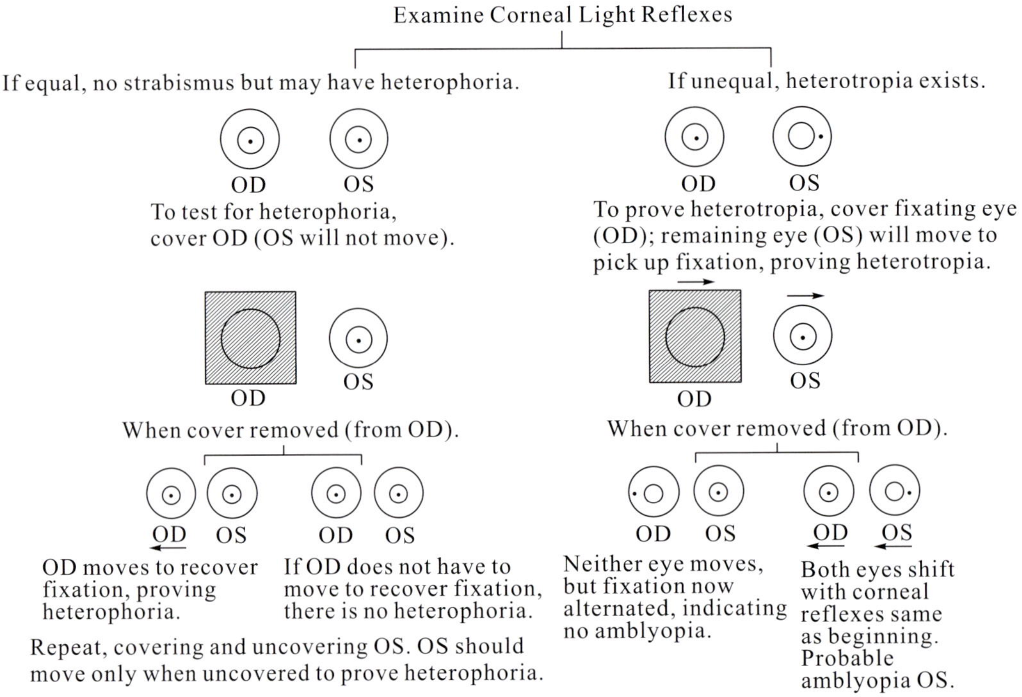

Examine Corneal Light Reflexes

If equal, no strabismus but may have heterophoria.

OD OS
To test for heterophoria, cover OD (OS will not move).

OD OS
When cover removed (from OD).

OD OS   OD OS
OD moves to recover fixation, proving heterophoria.   If OD does not have to move to recover fixation, there is no heterophoria.

Repeat, covering and uncovering OS. OS should move only when uncovered to prove heterophoria.

If unequal, heterotropia exists.

OD OS
To prove heterotropia, cover fixating eye (OD); remaining eye (OS) will move to pick up fixation, proving heterotropia.

OD OS
When cover removed (from OD).

OD OS   OD OS
Neither eye moves, but fixation now alternated, indicating no amblyopia.   Both eyes shift with corneal reflexes same as beginning. Probable amblyopia OS.

Figure 3-1 Cover test

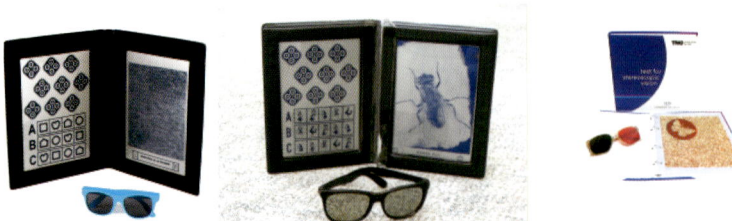

Figure 3-2 Stereopsis test

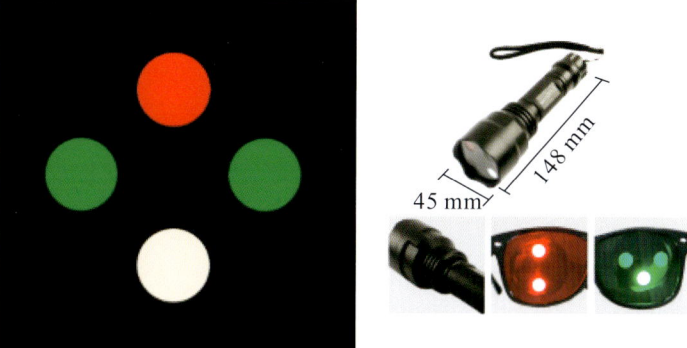

Figure 3-3 Worth 4-dot test

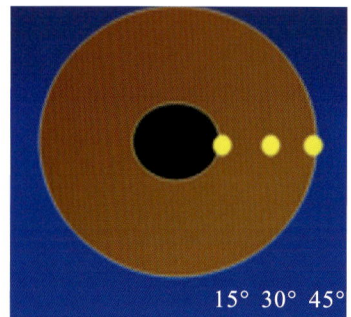

Figure 3-4 Hirschberg test

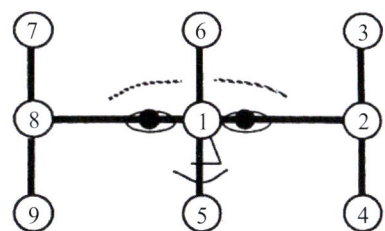

Figure 3-5 The sequential order of positions of gaze for EOM testing seen from the perspective of the examiner looking at the patient

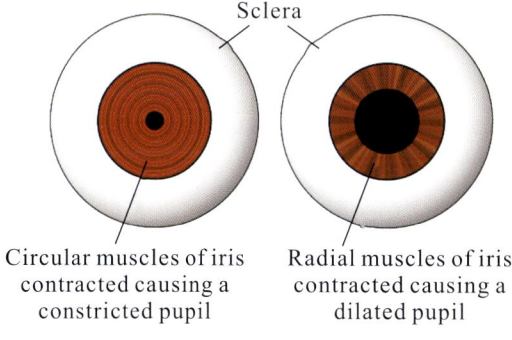

Figure 3-6 Pupillary reaction

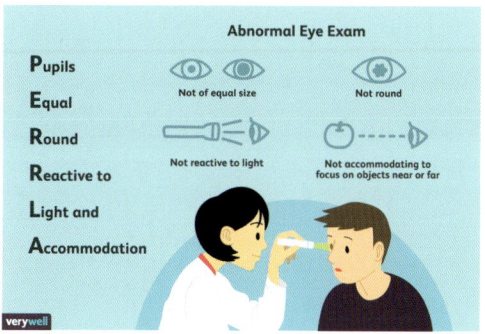

Figure 3-7 PERRLA

Chapter 5
Optics & Refraction

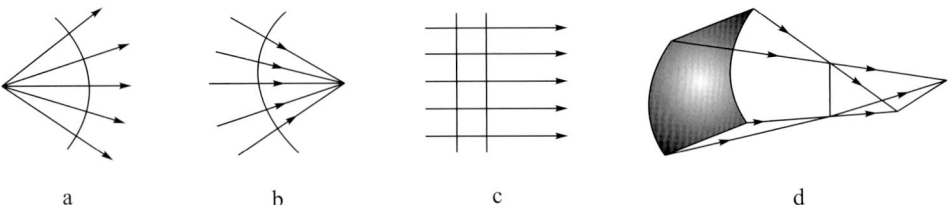

a. Convergent beams b. Divergent beams c. Parallel beams d. Astigmatic beams

Figure 5-1 Four types of beams

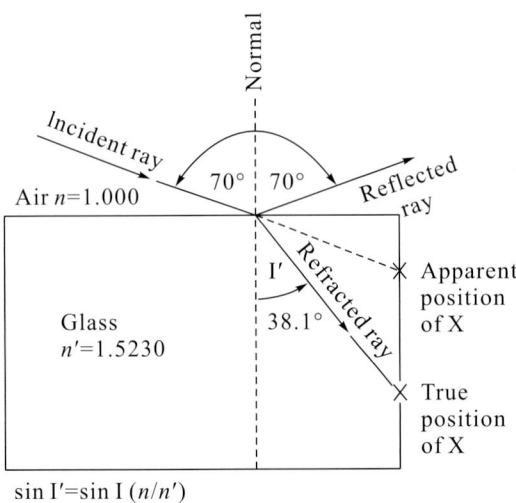

$\sin I' = \sin I \, (n/n')$

Figure 5-2 Reflection and refraction of light

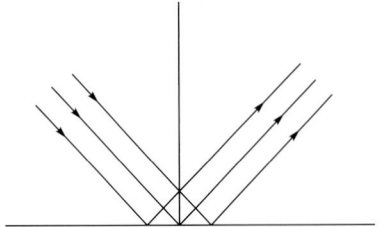

Figure 5-3 Specular reflection (Glossy surface)

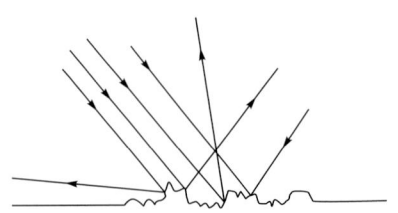

Figure 5-4 Diffusion (Rough surface)

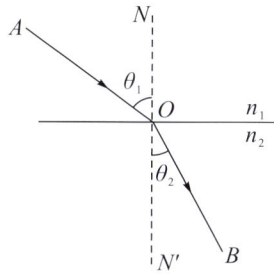
Figure 5-5 Laws of refraction

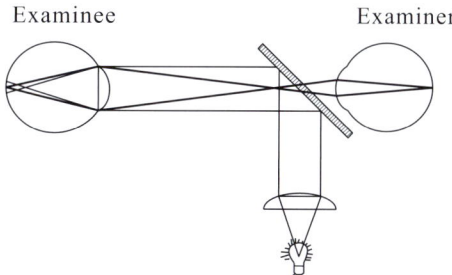
Figure 5-6 Retinoscopy principle

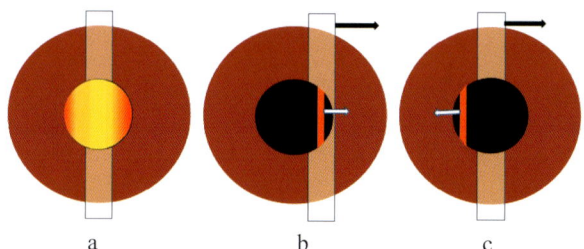

a. Neutralization point   b. With motion   c. Against motion

Figure 5-7 Red reflex during streak retinoscopy

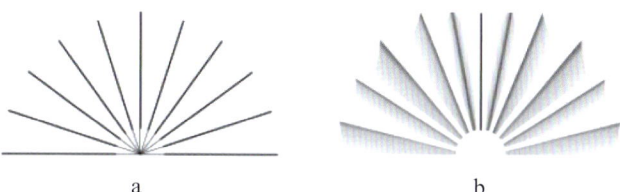

a. As seen by an emmetropic person   b. As seen by a patient with astigmatism at horizontal axis

Figure 5-8 Clock chart (Astigmatic fan)

Chapter 7
Spectacles

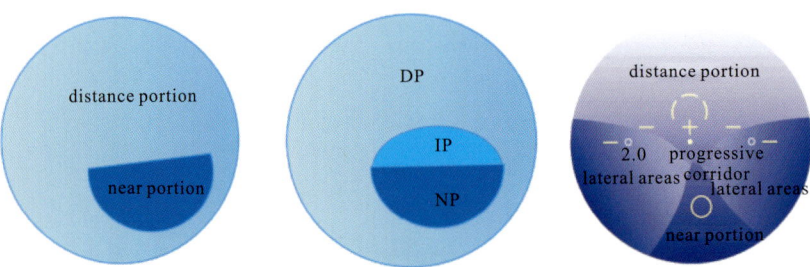

Figure 7-1 Bifocals, trifocals, and progressive multifocal lenses

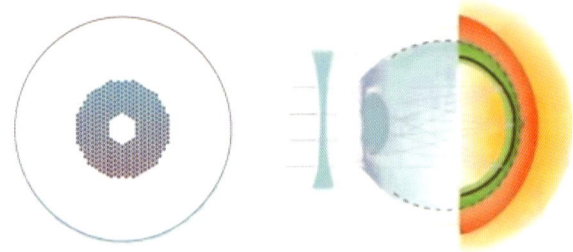

Figure 7-2 Peripheral defocus lenses

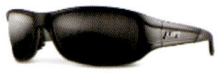 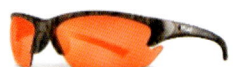 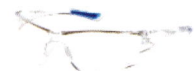

Figure 7-3 Safety glasses

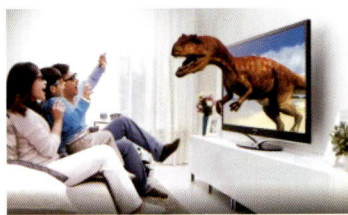

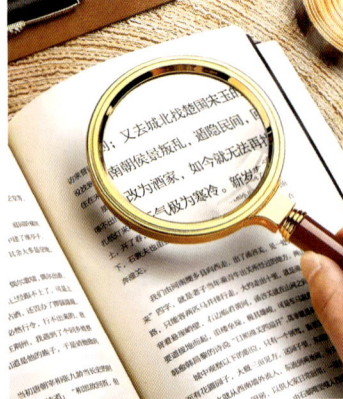

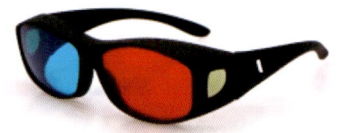

Figure 7-4 3D glasses

Figure 7-5 Magnifying lenses

Chapter 8
Contact Lenses

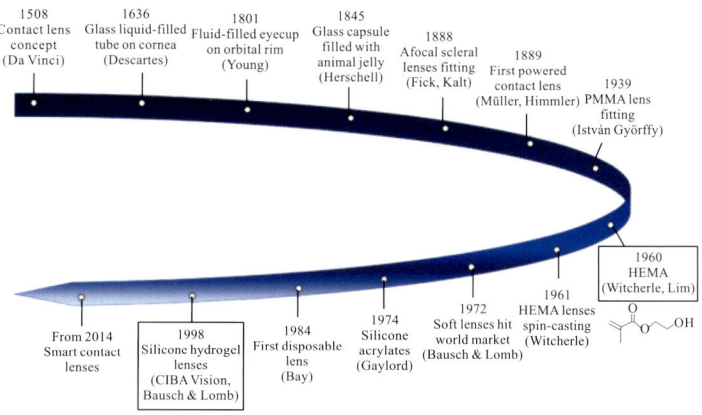

Figure 8-1 Timeline of contact lens evolution

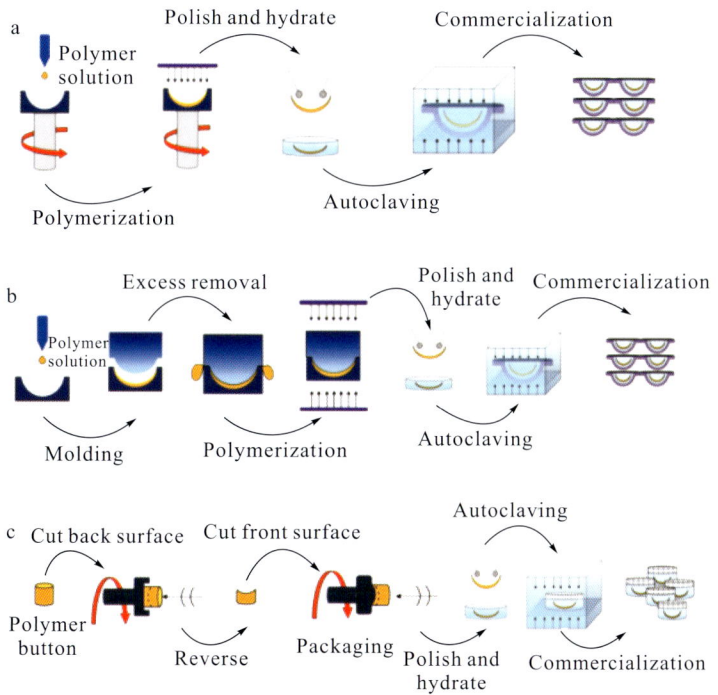

a. The spin casting process b. The injection molding process c. The lathe cutting process

Figure 8-2 Contact lens manufacturing process

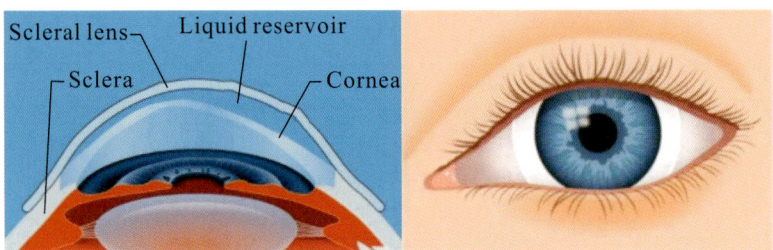

Figure 8-3 Scleral lens

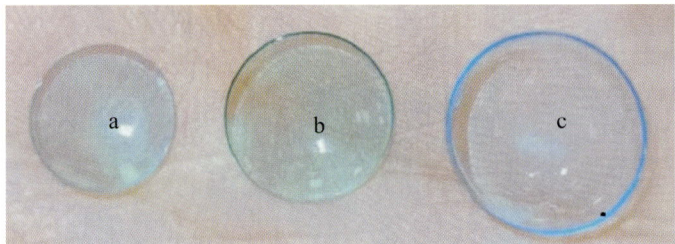

a. Rigid gas permeable lens(RGP)   b. Orthokeratology   c. Soft lens

Figure 8-4 Contact lens

Chapter 10
Glaucoma

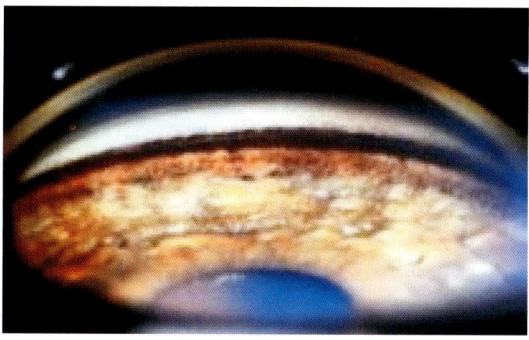

Figure 10-1 The angle structures of gonioscopic examination

Chapter 12
Lens Diseases

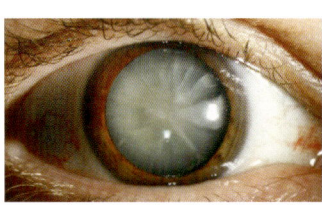

Figure 12-1　Cataract

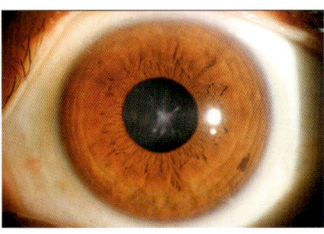

Figure 12-2　Congenital cataracts
（蓝色簇状混浊）

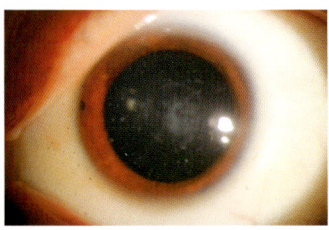

Figure 12-3　Congenital cataracts
（核性粉状混浊）

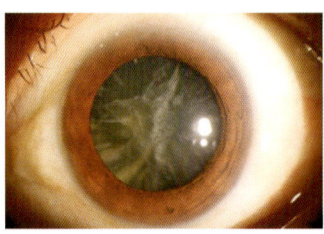

Figure 12-4　Cortical cataract,
incipient stage

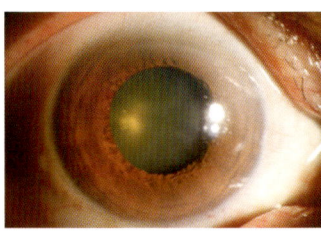

Figure 12-5　Immature stage

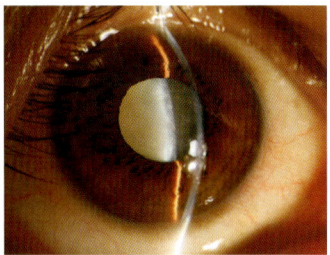

Figure 12-6　Mature stage

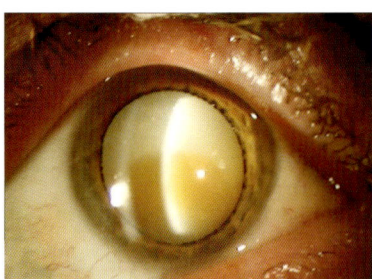

Figure 12-7　Hypermature stage

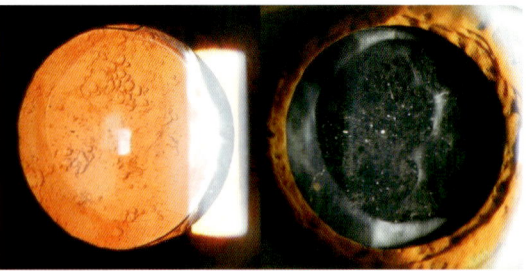

Figure 12-8　PCO

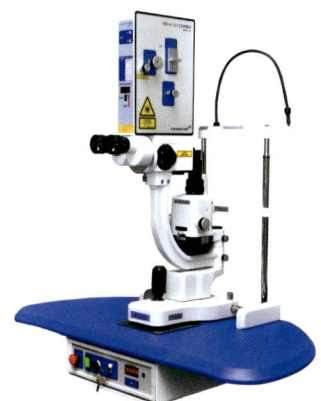

Figure 12-9 PCO treated with Nd:YAG laser

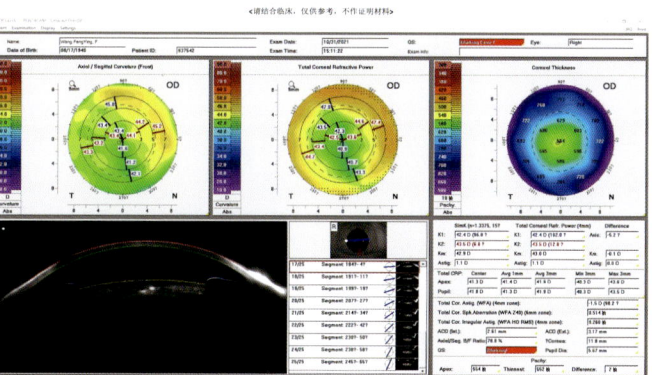

Figure 12-10 Pantacam

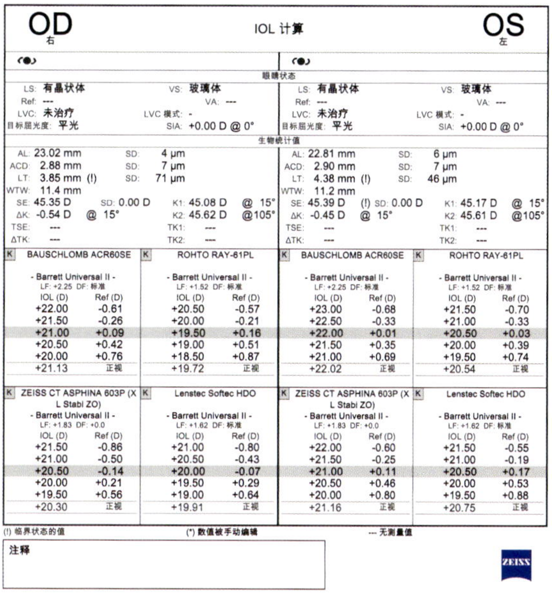

Figure 12-11 IOLmaster

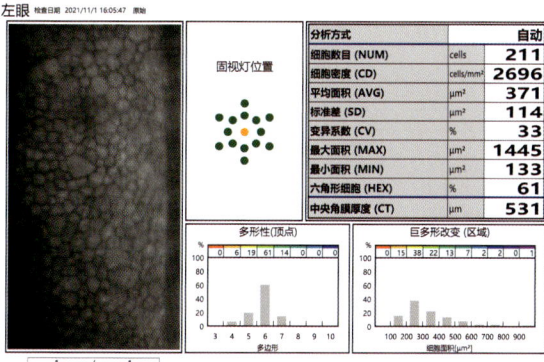

Figure 12-12 Corneal endothelial examination

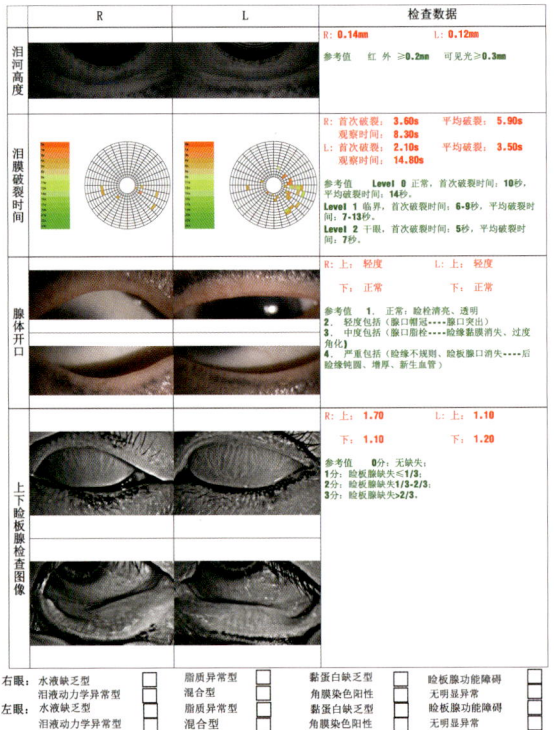

Figure 12-13 Ocular surface analyzer

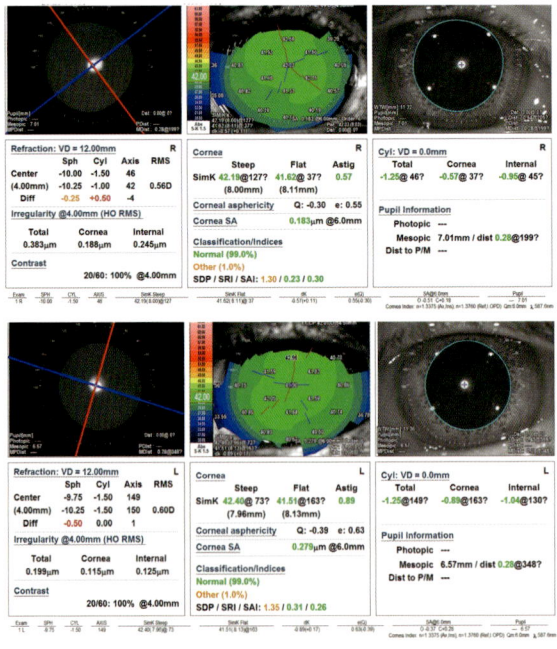

Figure 12-14 OPD

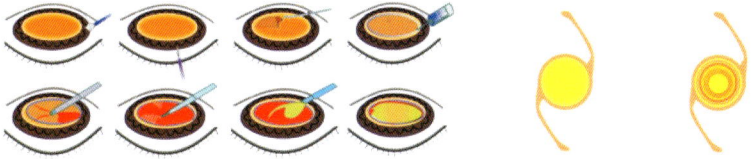

Figure 12-15 Phacoemulsification and the IOL

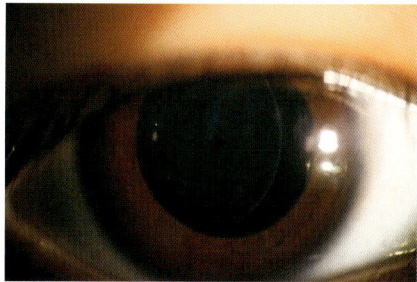

Figure 12-16 Lens subluxated in a patient with Marfan's syndrome

Chapter 17
Common Clinical Conversations

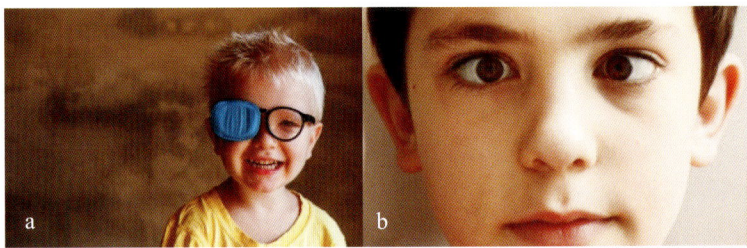

a. Amblyopia eye   b. Misaligned eye

Figure 17-1 Amblyopia eye and misaligned eye

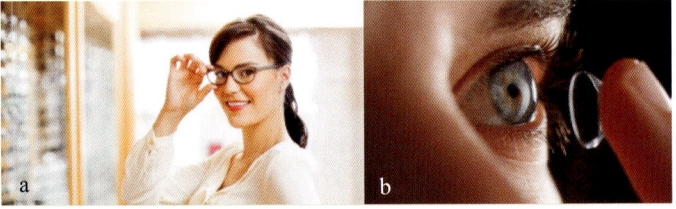

a. Wear glasses   b. Wear contact lenses

Figure 17-2 Wear glasses and wear contact lenses

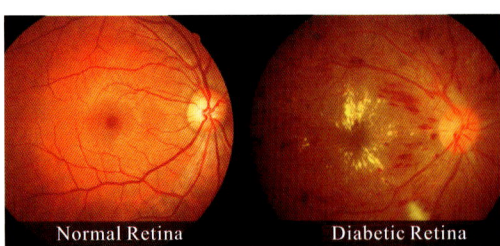

Figure 17-3 The fundus of diabetic

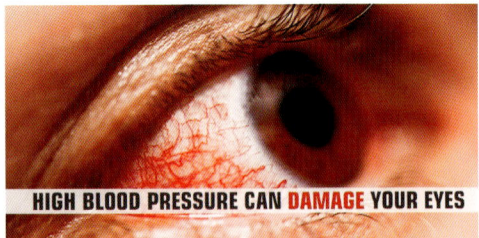

Figure 17-4 High blood pressure can damage eyes

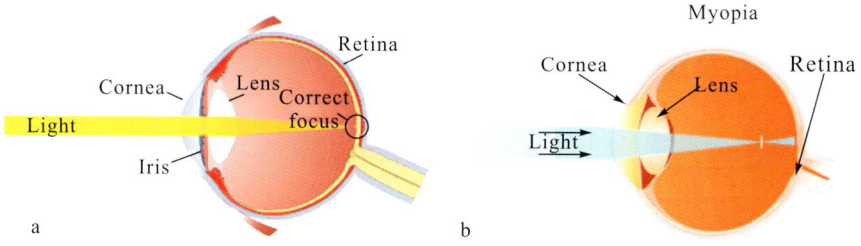

a. Normal condition   b. Myopia eye

Figure 17-5 Normal condition and myopia eye

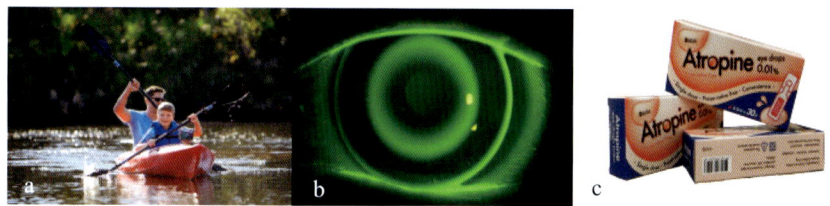

a. Outdoor activity   b. Orthokeratology   c. Atropine

Figure 17-6 Outdoor activity, orthokeratology and Atropine

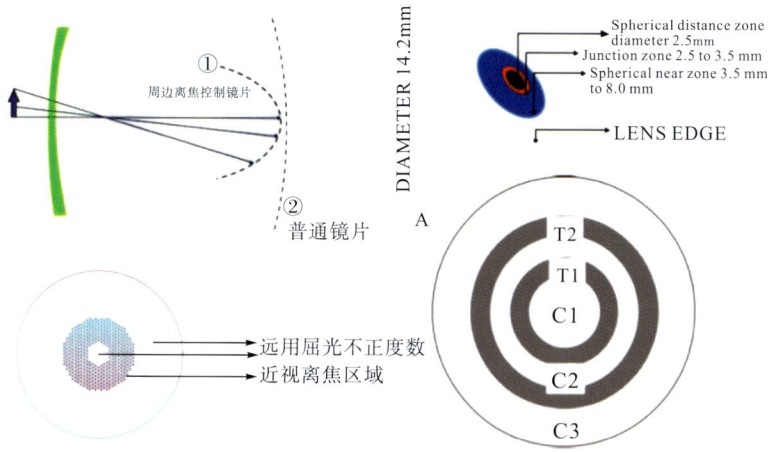

a. Peripheral defocus lenses   b. Soft defocus contact lenses

Figure 17-7 Peripheral defocus lenses and soft defocus contact lenses

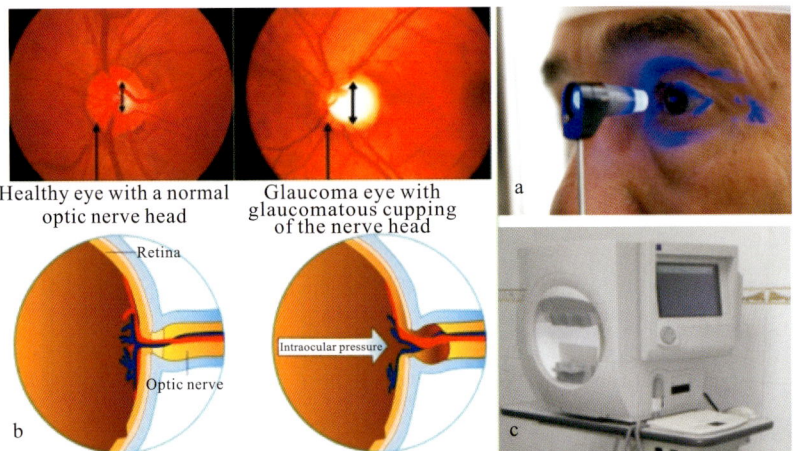

a. Intraocular pressure test   b. The C/D ratio   c. Visual field test

Figure 17-8 Intraocular pressure test, the C/D ratio and visual field test

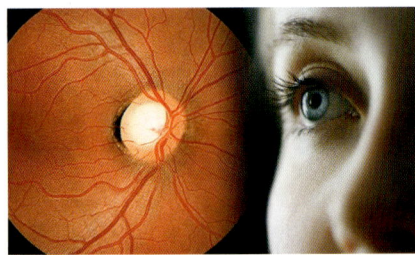

Figure 17-9 Glaucoma damages optic nerve fibers

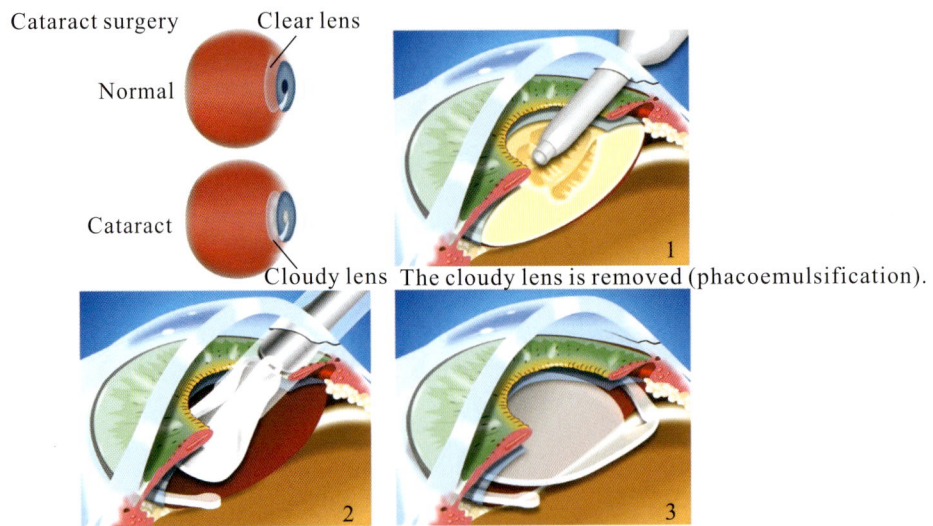

Figure 17-10 Cataract surgery procedure

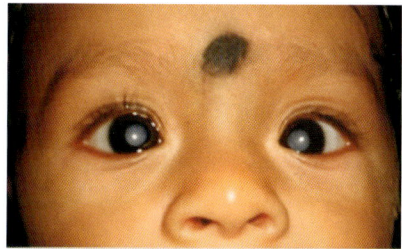

Figure 17-11 Infantile cataract

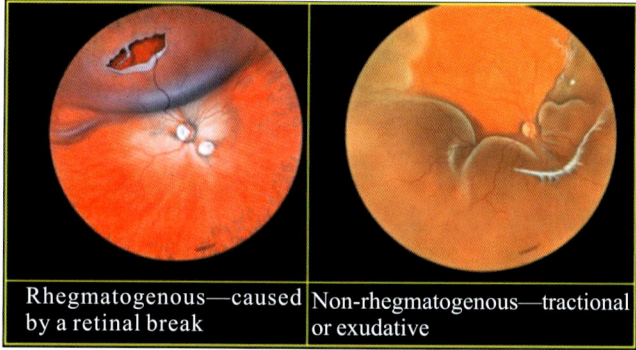

Figure 17-12 Types of retinal detachment

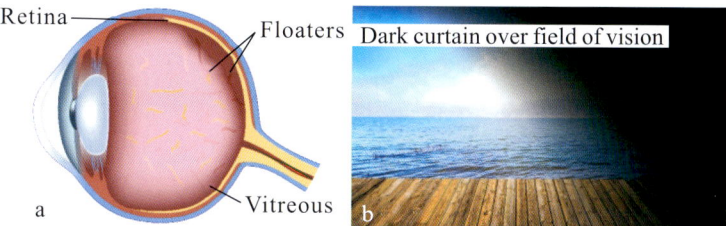

a. Floaters   b. Dark or curtain over field of vision

Figure 17-13 Symptoms of retinal detachment

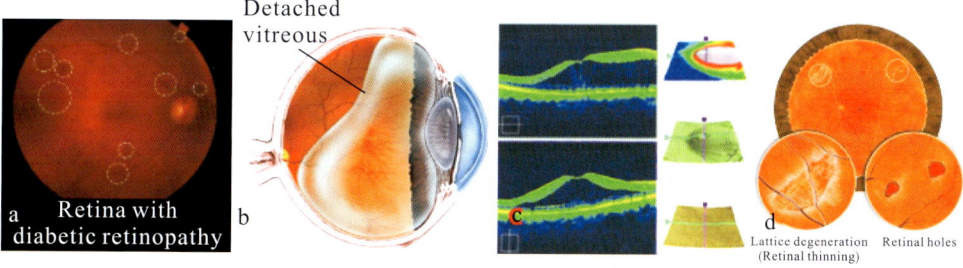

a. Diabetic retinopathy   b. Posterior vitreous detachment   c. Retinoschisis   d. Lattice degeneration

Figure 17-14 Some other problems with your eyes

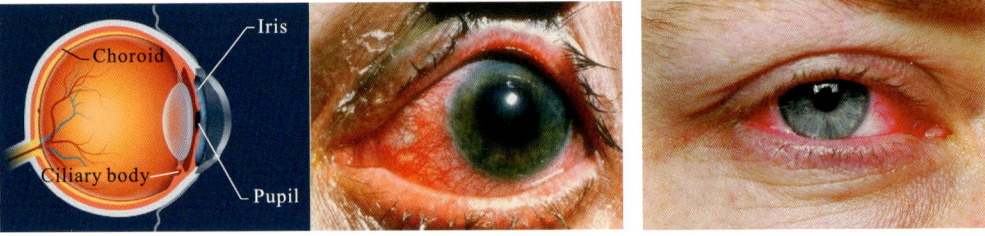

Figure 17-15 Iridocyclitis Figure 17-16 Conjunctivitis

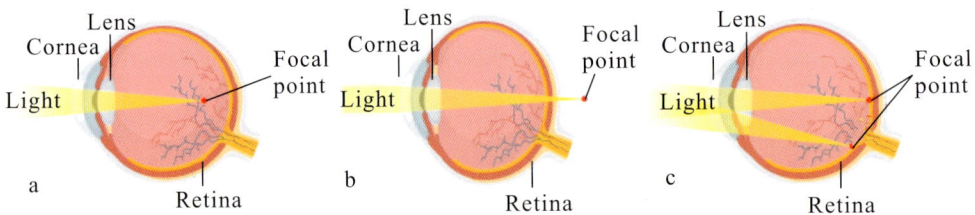

a. Myopia b. Hyperopia c. Astigmatism

Figure 17-17 Refractive errors

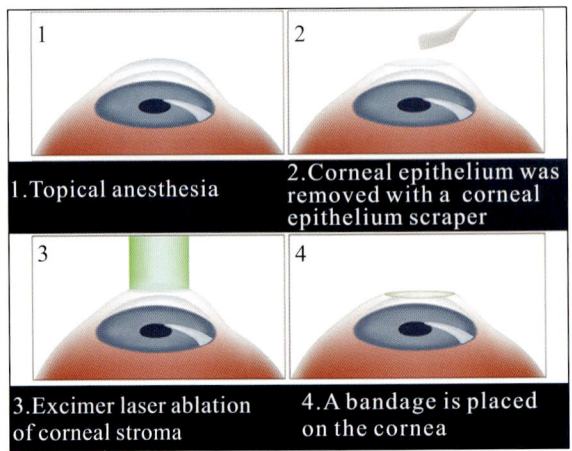

Figure 17-18 PRK surgery

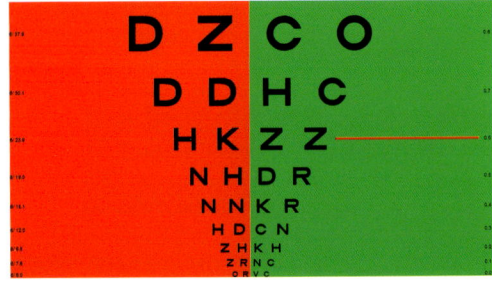

Figure 17-19 Duochrome balance visual target